I0055666

Living Related Transplantation

Living Related Transplantation

editors

Nadey Hakim
Ruben Canelo
Vassilios Papalois
Hammersmith Hospital London, UK

ICP

Imperial College Press

Published by

Imperial College Press
57 Shelton Street
Covent Garden
London WC2H 9HE

Distributed by

World Scientific Publishing Co. Pte. Ltd.
5 Toh Tuck Link, Singapore 596224
USA office: 27 Warren Street, Suite 401-402, Hackensack, NJ 07601
UK office: 57 Shelton Street, Covent Garden, London WC2H 9HE

British Library Cataloguing-in-Publication Data
A catalogue record for this book is available from the British Library.

LIVING RELATED TRANSPLANTATION

ISBN-13 978-1-84816-497-0
ISBN-10 1-84816-497-1

Typeset by Stallion Press
Email: enquiries@stallionpress.com

Printed in Singapore.

Contents

Contributors

Enrico Benedetti
Division of Transplant Surgery
Department of Surgery
University of Illinois at Chicago
840 S. Wood St. Suite #402 (M/C958)
Chicago, IL 60612, USA

Ruben Canelo
Department of Hepatobiliary and Pancreatic Surgery
Hammersmith Hospital
Imperial College London
Du Cane Road
London W12 0NN, UK

Hiroshi Date
Department of Thoracic Surgery
Kyoto University
54 Shogoin Kawahara-cho
Sakyo-ku, Kyoto 606-8507, Japan

Sheung Tat Fan
Department of Surgery
The University of Hong Kong
Queen Mary Hospital
102 Pokfulam Road
Hong Kong, China

Rainer Gruessner
Chairman, Department of Surgery
Professor of Surgery and Immunology
Arizona Health Sciences Center
1501 N. Campbell Avenue, Room 5408
P.O Box 245066
Tucson, AZ 85724-5066, USA

Nadey Hakim
Consultant Transplant and General Surgeon
Surgical Director of the Transplant Unit
St. Mary's NHS Trust
St. Mary's Hospital
Praed Street, Paddington
London W2 1NY, UK

Nicos Kessaris
Consultant Renal and Transplant Surgeon
Department of Renal Medicine and Transplantation
St. George's Hospital, Blackshaw Road
London SW17 0QT, UK

Chi Leung Liu
Department of Surgery
The University of Hong Kong
Queen Mary Hospital
Room 803, Central Building
1-3 Pedder Street, Central
Hong Kong, China

Evangelos Mazaris
West London Renal and Transplant Centre
Imperial College, Hammersmith Hospital
4th Floor Hammersmith House
London W12 0HS, UK

Nicola Morelli
Attending Surgeon, Department of Surgery
University of Illinois at Chicago
840-S. Wood Street, Chicago, IL 60612, USA

John Najarian
Transplant Center
University of Minnesota Medical Center
Phillips-Wangensteen Building
Second Floor, Clinic 2A
516 Delaware Street S.E.
Minneapolis, MN 55455, USA

Eduardo Olavarria
Medical Director – BMT Programme
Haematology Department
Hospital de Navarra
Irunlarrea 3
Pamplona 31008, Spain

Fabrizio Panaro
Transplant Fellow, Department of Surgery
University of Illinois at Chicago
840-S. Wood Street, Chicago, IL 60612, USA

Vassilios Papalois
West London Renal and Transplant Centre
Imperial College, Hammersmith Hospital
4th Floor Hammersmith House
London W12 0HS, UK

Nobuyoshi Shimizu
Department of Cancer and Thoracic Surgery
Okayama University
2-5-1 Shikata-cho
Okayama 700-8558, Japan

David Sutherland
Professor and Head, Division of Transplantation
Director, Schulze Diabetes Institute
Department of Surgery, University of Minnesota
420 Delaware Street SE, MMC 280; 11-200 PWB
Minneapolis, MN 55455, USA

Giuliano Testa
Associate Professor of Surgery
Director, Liver Transplantation and Hepatobiliary Surgery
Center for Advanced Medicine, University of Chicago
5758 S. Maryland Avenue, Chicago, IL 60637, USA

Foreword

Living donor kidney transplantation was first performed in Paris in 1953 by Jean Hamburger and his team. The development of renal transplantation as a clinical field over the next 20 years was highly dependent on the use of live donor kidneys. During most of these two decades, organs from deceased donors could be obtained only after cessation of heartbeat and respiration. Consequently, observations in recipients of the ischemically compromised deceased donor grafts were so variable that definitive conclusions about immunosuppression and tissue typing were reached primarily by studies of live donor kidney recipients.

Live kidney donation was no secret and aroused surprisingly little negative reaction from the public. It was, however, a divisive issue within the medical profession because live donation potentially placed healthy people in harm's way and therefore appeared to violate the deep-rooted tradition of *primum non nocere* (first do no harm). It was essential to develop agreement within the medical profession on the probity of the practice. A kidney-specific consensus about living donor transplantation was reached by the early 1970s following a series of ethical-medical conferences and publications.

A seminal question from the beginning was 'what conceivable benefit was there for the previously healthy live donor?' A defensible way out was found at the ethics conferences and in law courts with the argument that the fullness of the donor's emotional life and welfare was often dependent on that of the recipient. Under these circumstances, the long-term benefits to the donor could be viewed in many cases as equivalent to those of the recipient. This was most frequently obvious when the transplantation was between family members. In addition, it began to be argued by the mid-1980s that live kidney donation had to be considered in the context of society's needs.

In the social context, emerging pivotal problems had been caused by a rapidly growing but unmet need for transplantable kidneys; a long list of transplant candidates on long-term dialysis were waiting in vain for organs. At an administrative level, the fiscal viability of transplant centres frequently depended on a supply of live donor organs. It was feared that closure of the handmaiden transplant programmes would inhibit the homogeneous diffusion of end-stage renal disease care into national health care systems. From the perspective of 'group ethics', it was argued by some that the death of one volunteer per 2000 donations was a statistical non-event in relation to the life years saved.

In more recent times, the use of live donor kidneys has increased dramatically, while the concept of volunteer donation has extended to the liver and other non-renal organs. Support for live-donor liver transplantation (LDLT) was built on the same ethical-social base as kidney transplantation by regulatory and oversight committees at the University of Chicago. Publication of the Chicago LDLT proposal in a 1989 issue of the *New England Journal of Medicine* helped launch LDLT programs that revolutionised the treatment of children with biliary atresia and other hepatic disorders.

At first, LDLT was employed mainly in Asian centres, where deceased donation did not exist, and was used almost entirely for the treatment of children. By the mid-1990s, however, LDLT for adults was begun. Worldwide experience in various liver donor operations rapidly accumulated until it was recognised that the donor mortality was many times greater than that of kidney donations, and that the highest donor risk was with right lobar LDLTs. Inevitably, other kinds of non-renal living donor transplantation have emerged: pancreas, lung and intestine.

It is apparent that non-renal live donor organ transplantation is on the same developmental path as that of blood transfusion in the first half of the 20th century, and kidney and stem cell transplantation in the last half. With the kidney and the non-renal organ procedures, the principal concern has been the physical and emotional health risk to the live donor. The risk–benefit ratio, as this applies to both donors and recipients, has yet to be finalised for living donor liver, lung, pancreas (or islet) and intestinal transplantation.

In this text, the editors have compiled a series of chapters about all these procedures. Because the chapters were written by pioneer proponents of the different kinds of transplantation, the resulting slender book has the weight of authority, and will be a valuable resource to anyone interested in developing a global view of the ethics and practice of transplantation.

Thomas E. Starzl
University of Pittsburgh School of Medicine

Chapter 1

Ethical Issues in Living Donor Transplantation

Vassilios Papalois and Evangelos Mazaris

Introduction

Live-donor transplantation is an amazing act of altruism that affects the lives of the donor, the recipient and their families forever. Some of the greatest triumphs of modern surgery are associated with live donor transplantation. All of them are characterized by a lot of inspired and tremendously hard work of multidisciplinary medical teams and the courage and determination of the patients and their families.

Live-donor kidney transplantation is the treatment of choice for end-stage renal failure. The main reasons for this are as follows: (a) the transplant is performed when the donor and the recipient are in an optimum medical condition and at a time that is convenient for them and their families, (b) recipients of live-donor kidney grafts enjoy much better long-term graft survival and quality of life compared to recipients of cadaveric kidney grafts,[1–3] (c) it reduces the cost for the health service for every patient with end-stage renal failure, since the cost of dialysis (£60,000/patient/year) is substituted by the cost of live-donor kidney transplant (£25,000/patient), adding the cost of the immunosuppressive medications, (£3,000/patient/year) and (d) it reduces the number of patients on the cadaveric waiting list and therefore increases the chances of patients with no potential live donor to be transplanted. This is particularly important since the gap between the number of cadaveric donors and the number of patients on the waiting list is increasing. This can be explained partly by the development of strong national campaigns for safe driving, a significant improvement in the safety features of vehicles (e.g. airbags) and a more stringent monitoring by the police which have caused a reduction in road-traffic accidents, as well as an introduction of healthier lifestyles, which has led to the reduction of strokes. In the UK, data from UK Transplant, the national regulatory authority for organ donation and transplantation, demonstrated that between 1994 and 2003, there was an increase of 60.1% of the patients on the cadaveric list for kidney transplant and a 16.7% decrease in the number of cadaveric donors.[4] In fact, there is a growing population of patients maintained on dialysis all over the world, while the number of donors fails to meet such demand or is even decreasing as has happened in the UK (Fig. 1). Although there is an increase in the number of live-donor kidney transplants in the UK (18% from 2002 to 2003, 372 to 439 respectively), still there is a long way to go and the number remains lower compared to the Scandinavian countries, which have the higher percentage of live kidney donors in Europe (Table 1).

Similarly, over the last two decades live-donor transplants are being performed very successfully for other solid organs, such as the lung (total or lobe), liver (lobe or lobes), pancreas (only its tail) and part of the small bowel. This is seen especially in countries such as Japan or India, where cadaveric donation is limited by religious and cultural prohibitions against the concept of brain death, and live donors may be the only source of organs for transplantation.

Retrieving an organ or part of an organ from an otherwise healthy individual and exposing them to the risks of surgery (however safe it might be in experienced hands and in modern transplant centres) as well as to the potential long-term risks for their health and quality of life, for the benefit of another person, posses several ethical questions that have initiated a great deal of medical and public debate.

Ethical Issues

Safety

The first issue is the safety of the surgical removal of organs from an otherwise healthy individual; what are the long-term consequences of living, for example, with one kidney and what is the effect of such a procedure on

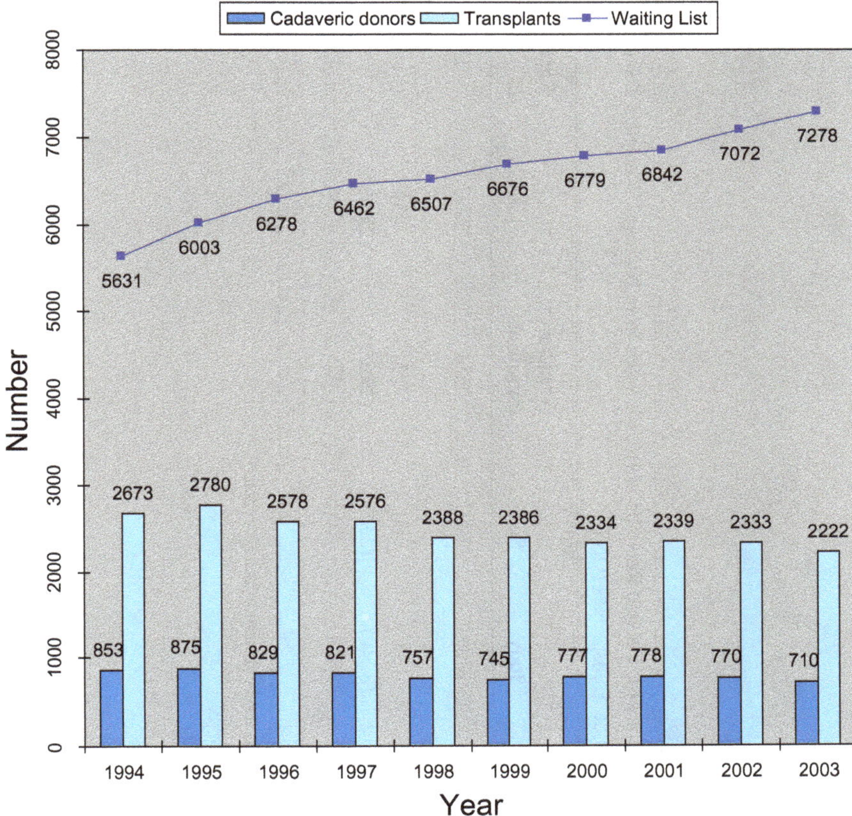

Figure 1: Number of cadaveric donors and kidney transplants in the UK and patients on the waiting list for the period 1994–2003. Obtained from UK Transplant showing the decrease in cadaveric donors and the increase in patients on the waiting list for a kidney transplant from 1994 to 2003.

quality of life? Undoubtedly the risks for living donors of segmental liver, segmental lung and segmental pancreas transplants are greater. The mortality rate of live-donor nephrectomy has been calculated to be 0.03%[5] with the life expectancy of a live kidney donor similar to that of the general population.[6,7] Many surveys have reported excellent quality of life for live donors[8–12] and a meta-analysis of the minority who exhibited negative feelings regarding donation demonstrated that they had donated to recipients

Table 1: Kidney transplant activity in Europe, 2003. Figures for UK and Republic of Ireland taken from National Transplant Database, March 2004 and all others from the Organizacion Nacional de Transplantes (ONT).

	Eurotransplant[a]	France	Italy	Spain	Scandia[b] transplant	UK	Republic of Ireland
Cadaveric kidney transplants	3345	1991	1489	1991	654	1297	133
Live-donor kidney transplants	646 (16.2%)	136 (6.4%)	135 (8.3%)	60 (2.9%)	271 (29.3%)	439 (25.3%)	0
Total kidney transplants	3991	2127	1624	2051	925	1736	133

[a] Eurotransplant includes Germany, Austria, Belgium, Luxembourg, the Netherlands and Slovenia.
[b] Scandia Transplant includes Denmark, Norway, Finland and Sweden.

who died within one year after the procedure. Although animal studies demonstrated that glomerular hyperfiltration in the remaining kidney could eventually compromise its function, it was proven by several studies in humans, with a follow-up period of over 20 years, that the remaining kidney did not present any functional abnormality[13,14] apart from a slight increase in the rate of proteinuria but with no clinical significance.[15] The longest presented follow-up of people with one kidney was a 45-year follow-up survey of 62 World War II veterans, who had undergone uninephrectomy after renal trauma, yet their survival rate was similar to that of other veterans.[16]

There are three types of operations for a live-donor nephrectomy: the classic open nephrectomy with a wide flank incision, laparoscopic nephrectomy using key-hole surgery and the mini-open nephrectomy with a small loin incision of 8 ± 1 cm anterior to the eleventh rib without rib resection and with the use of laparoscopic instruments.[17] The classic open operation may act as a disincentive for the donor because of increased surgical pain, increased hospital stay, poor cosmetic result and extended period of convalescence. With the introduction of minimally invasive techniques the surgical morbidity has decreased, there is earlier return to normal daily activities as well as work and the cosmetic outcome is excellent. In the beginning, laparoscopic nephrectomy was considered as harmful because of longer warm ischaemia time (the period lasting from the clamping of the renal vessels until perfusion of the retrieved kidney with cold preservation solution), but with the advent of modern devices (e.g. endocatch) that period was shortened making it comparable to open nephrectomy.[18] In a survey it was demonstrated that, although the introduction of laparoscopic nephrectomy influenced positively potential recipients, probably because they anticipated minimal complication inflicted upon their donors, it had less impact on potential donors' decision to donate.[19] However, in laparoscopic donor nephrectomy there is an increased incidence of ureteral complications and the pneumoperitoneum decreases renal cortical blood flow and urine output.[20,21] The mini-open nephrectomy technique offers the advantages of laparoscopic nephrectomy and it also reduces warm ischaemia and operating times, making it even safer for the potential donor.[17] Even life insurance companies in the US have acknowledged the above facts and in a conducted survey 94% of them do not consider the otherwise healthy donor to be at increased risk of morbidity or mortality after donating, yet only 2% would increase the premium for such a donor.[22]

Donor's motivation

Another important ethical issue is the motivation of the donor. From recent surveys[23,24] several categories of motives for live-organ donors have been identified.

First of all there is a desire to help, which is very strong and often considered as something natural. Another is a feeling of moral duty, that is, in order to distinguish it from the desire to help, a perception that donation is something that you are expected to do. The majority of donors derive a tremendous degree of satisfaction and an increase in their self-esteem from doing good deeds. Also, some donors may imagine themselves in the recipient's situation, especially siblings, who are sure that the latter would act accordingly if they were in a similar state. Furthermore, spouses may be motivated by self-benefit from their companion's improved health and the improvement of the couple's quality of life. That may be the case for parents as well, together with the feeling of moral duty. A minority may feel coercion to donate especially by other family members fearing that relations among family members would be disturbed if they denied donation. There may be several factors in support of donation and others causing concern (Table 2). More rare motives may be religious beliefs or a feeling of guilt in past relationships.

Donor's feelings about donation

The decision to donate is, psychologically, a complicated one. For example, potential emotionally related donors are informed that dialysis is an alternative option and therefore kidney transplantation is not a life-saving procedure, yet still they feel that they are the only option for the potential recipient.[24] Another important result from a recent survey in Scandinavia is that males regard donation as an extraordinary gift, whereas females regard it as an extension of family obligations.[23] Another particular aspect of the concept of donation is that the decision to donate is spontaneous and usually donors do not experience negative consequences regarding

Table 2: Several factors work in support of the motives and the decision to donate. Other factors are of concern but did not prevent the respondents from donating.[24]

Factors in Support

- Previous knowledge of transplantation and donation.
- Long-standing awareness of the relative's future need of a transplant.
- Getting a good health screening during assessment.
- The long waiting time for a cadaveric kidney transplant.
- Trust in the health care services.
- Support from family and friends.
- Recognition from the recipient.
- Oral and written information.

Factors of Concern

- Fear of not passing the medical screening.
- Fear of surgery and long-term consequences.
- Fear of poor outcome for the recipient.
- Objections in the family.
- Concern that alternative potential donors have not come forward.
- Weak emotional relationship with the recipient.

family relationships, with conflicts between the donor and the family being rare.[25] However, in order not to affect the sensitive family relationships, the transplant team should achieve the wider possible family consensus regarding the donor's decision to donate thus minimizing the possibility of any future conflicts. It has also been demonstrated by various surveys that the majority of donors would have made the same choice again without regretting their decision[26,27] and would even encourage others to donate.[12] According to other surveys, although parents decide immediately to donate there is a degree of ambivalence experienced by some fathers.[28] In the same study it was demonstrated that the decision for siblings is more complex and may cause conflict between family of birth and family of marriage.

Recipient's feelings about donation

For the recipients, feelings of guilt are more prominent especially if they have a close relationship with the donor.[29] An interesting study showed that adolescent recipients of parental grafts experienced strong feeling of obligation and debt, which led to psychological distress, and social as well as familial alienation, probably because of the enhancement of the usual parent–adolescent conflict due to the transplant procedure.[28] However, other studies[30] did not demonstrate a negative impact on family relations in parent-to-child donation, taking into consideration that the children of this study were younger and not adolescents. It is also interesting that recipients are sometimes reluctant to accept a live-donor kidney when offered to them, and as a study confirmed, more than half of the patients on dialysis declined the offer of a live-donor kidney because of concerns about the donor's health and fearing also that the procedure would compromise their relationship with the donor.[31]

Donor approach, consent and evaluation

Prior to accepting a potential donor, every effort has to be made to ensure that their offer is genuine and voluntary. The person who consents to be a live donor should be 'competent, willing to donate, free from coercion, medically and psychosocially suitable, fully informed of the risks, benefits and alternative treatment available to the recipient'.[32] The most important elements of informed consent are: (a) understanding, (b) medical and psychological suitability, (c) the process of informing the donor, (d) absence of coercion and free choice, and (e) documentation of consent.

The potential donors have the right to receive and understand all the necessary information (Table 3) regarding the risks and benefits to themselves as well as the alternative treatments that could be offered to the potential recipient. The source of such information is essential and certainly could not come, for example, from brochures or the recipient's physician, as a recent study demonstrated.[23] Transplant centres seem to be the potential donor's only source of information since they possess the relative scientific experience to inform him. Yet a transplant centre may have a number of reasons for wanting an organ donation to go ahead: transplants are their source of income; they are able to increase their prestige and conduct research but they may also display a strong desire to help the recipient. Negative information should be presented to the donor. This might have a negative effect, but that is why the transplant team should

Table 3: Information elements for potential living donors (live-organ donor consensus group).[32]

- Description of the evaluation, the surgical procedure and the recuperative period.
- Anticipated short- and long-term follow-up care.
- Alternative donation procedures even if only available at other transplant centres.
- Potential surgical complications for the donor, citing the reports of donor deaths (even if never experienced at that transplant centre).
- Medical uncertainties, including the potential for long-term donor complications.
- Any expenses to be borne by the donor.
- Potential impact of donation on the ability of the donor to obtain health and life insurance.
- Potential impact of donation on the lifestyle of the donor and the ability to obtain future employment.
- Information regarding specific risks and benefits to the potential recipient.
- Expected outcome of transplantation for the recipient.
- Any alternative treatments (other than organ replacement) available to the recipient.
- Transplant centre-specific statistics of donor and recipient outcomes.

inform the donor meticulously[33] so that they can make a truly voluntary decision. For these reasons, independent donor counsellors are required with experience in issues related to live-donor transplantation and medical ethics. Others[1] have advocated that the first approach to the potential donor should come from the potential recipient and not from the latter's physician or surgeon, although they could offer their assistance in order to facilitate this process. The fact that more education is needed regarding live-donor kidney transplantation is also demonstrated by studies showing that the public may exhibit unrealistic fears regarding the issue, which may act as a disincentive for donation.[34,35] Probably the best way to assess if a potential donor has been adequately informed is whether they are surprised by anything that happens after consent is given.[32]

All potential donors should be screened for psychological and emotional stability and warned about possible psychosocial impairment that might occur in the postoperative period.[36] Psychosis or substance abuse might hinder the provision of effective operative and postoperative care, thus, leading to exclusion of such candidates for donation. Moreover, social evaluation of the potential donor is also necessary since financial hardship and marital problems, which indicate social instability, may cause several problems. The person who will make the psychosocial evaluation of the potential donor should be a trained psychologist or psychiatrist.

The argument that the potential donors require a lot of information and thinking prior to deciding to donate is, according to some studies, a myth.[37] A quick decision to donate is valid, despite the fact that it might not be fully informed, since rapid offers made by close relatives seem to be genuine and ethically acceptable in spite of incomplete understanding of what is involved.[38] However, adequate information should always be provided to the potential donor as well as establishing that it is understood. A characteristic example is that for many parents it is crucial, as well as adequate, to be aware that their child is ill and they could help by donating a kidney. This does not mean that the effort to inform the potential donor has to be abandoned, but in cases where the potential donor and recipient are close and sentimentally related, rapid or instant decision making should not invalidate consent. Nor should the donor, under any circumstances, be sacrificed for the recipient even if they are prepared to accept the sacrifice; that is why an offer by a prisoner to donate his second kidney to his daughter, after having donated his other kidney again to her a few years ago, was declined.[39]

Many of the potential donors may feel obligated to donate to their emotionally related recipients and they may feel unable to have true freedom of choice. Someone could argue how anyone could deny donation when the lives of close relatives are at stake? Moral and emotional commitments are not constraints of freedom but are rather a part of ordinary human life.[40] On the other hand, we should wonder how could anyone face their family members if they deny donation? That is why an independent experienced psychologist should establish that the potential donor is free from coercion and external pressure. The donor should also be given a certain period of time to review the decision to donate as well as the liberty to withdraw at any point of the evaluation process. Some[41] believe that the reluctant donor should be provided with a medical alibi to justify his hesitation to the family. However, the general belief is that physicians should always be truthful and clear to their patients, avoiding lying and falsifying medical documents, which can clearly have catastrophic consequences.

Donor/transplant team's autonomy

It seems that the general public strongly believe that it is the donor's sole right to donate an organ and this decision should rest with the donor.[42] Yet, for physicians the prevailing principle according to the Hippocratic Oath is to 'do no harm'. Does a surgeon have an obligation to remove a person's organ upon request? In liberal and democratic societies everyone has the right to participate in dangerous activities according to their will, but the transplant procedure involves an 'accomplice'; the transplant surgeon. Rejection of a potential donor by the transplant surgeon may seem a paternalistic act, yet physicians are also responsible for the potential donor's welfare and should act in what they believe is their best interest. Despite the low donor mortality and morbidity rate, the transplant surgeon always risks causing harm to an otherwise healthy person. It is unethical for physicians to conduct harmful interventions and create medical problems deliberately such as in the aforementioned example of the father-prisoner who wanted to donate his remaining kidney to his daughter.[39] If transplant physicians feel unable to accept a potential donor they should inform them of the reasons for rejection as well as offer them referral for a second opinion. A transplant surgeon may refuse to accept a donor because of: (a) a borderline medical problem (e.g. borderline hypertension) that may aggravate after donation); (b) elderly donors and (c) potential serious technical difficulties during the operation that might increase the risk of complications.

Many donors are rejected because of advanced age, although one may wonder, is it physical or biological age that counts? Donors may argue that it is upon them to decide whether to undertake the increased risk. What if a mother at added risk wants to donate to her child whose health is deteriorating, even though donation is considered by the transplant centre ill-advised?[43] Should the determination of acceptability, in such cases, rest with the transplant centre alone? There are great variations in the exclusion criteria used by various transplant centres.[6] Because of these differences in the exclusion criteria (Table 4) research is required, concerning results on the outcome of increased risk donations, in order to achieve a consensus either on the aforementioned criteria or even on the way to introduce them.

Table 4: Acceptance and exclusion criteria for living donors at US transplant centres.[6]

Risk factor	Centres accepting (%)
History of renal stones	56
Microhaematuria	56
Alcohol abuse	89
Heroin and cocaine abuse	66
Risk factor	**Centres excluding (%)**
GFR < 80 ml/min/1.73m^2	59
GFR < 60 ml/min/1.73m^2	80
All patients with proteinuria	58
Some patients with proteinuria	90
Moderate obesity	16
Heavy cigarette use	16
Family history of type II diabetes	17
Type II diabetes	88–90

It has been suggested that donor's age ≥ 55 years negatively affected the 1- and 5-year kidney graft survival rate.[44,45] Other researchers have not found any difference in graft survival according to the age of the donor.[46] Grafts from older donors may display tissue inflammation at the time of procurement which may increase immune recognition.[47] There are changes associated with age in the number and size of glomeruli in nephrons, a progressive decrease in glomerular filtration rate as well as increased immunogenicity of the aging kidney. This data seems to contradict those who advocate that physical age does not count and biological age of the donor should be the criterion to proceed with the transplant.

Furthermore, there is debate on the length of time that a patient suffering from renal failure should remain on dialysis. Studies have proved that an increased time on dialysis has a negative effect on graft[48] and recipient survival.[49] It is probable that the reasons are the longer history of end-stage renal disease with the accumulation of co-morbid conditions as well as the increase in the rate of acute rejection through various immunological mechanisms.[50,51] Researchers also found that pre-emptive transplantation i.e. transplantation before exposure to any period of dialysis, was associated with better graft survival when compared to transplantation performed after the initiation of dialysis.[52–54] Although in an initial study the short duration of dialysis >6 months worsened graft survival but not patient survival,[52] in a more recent study it was demonstrated that the worsening of the graft outcome only became significant after six months on dialysis, whereas the recipient survival was significantly worsened only after one year on dialysis.[55] These facts could support those who advocate that we should allow the patient with end-stage renal disease to remain on dialysis for a limited period of time, in order to become aware of the advantages and disadvantages of such treatment and compare it with the patient's quality of life after transplantation, so that they can appreciate it more.

Live unrelated donation

It has been well established that live unrelated (i.e. emotionally related donors such as spouses, partners or friends) kidney grafts have better long-term survival than cadaveric ones and are comparable to live related grafts.[56–58] In the US, in 1987, spouses accounted for 2% of living kidney donors, yet by 1997 they accounted for almost 10% (Fig. 2). In a 1996 survey in the US, 90% of transplant centres accepted emotionally related donors and 60% encouraged emotionally related donation, 40% of them preferring spouses and only 21% accepting friends, demonstrating a marked change in attitudes compared to a similar survey performed in 1989.[59] Advocates of spousal donation from the US,[59,60] Japan[61] and Switzerland[62] have reported improved family psychodynamics including strengthening of marital bond, restoration of the functional role of the husband and wife, improved sexual relationship and emotional bonding with children. On the other hand, in certain cultures where the male is a dominant figure, spouses may be forced to donate. That is why spousal donation remains illegal in France[63] and involves complex procedures in the UK.[64] In the UK, the Unrelated Live Transplant Regulatory Authority (ULTRA) assesses the ethical and moral issues in proposed transplants between genetically unrelated individuals requiring both potential donor and recipient to write personal statements as part of the procedure. There are propositions for its abolition[65] because spousal donation is becoming

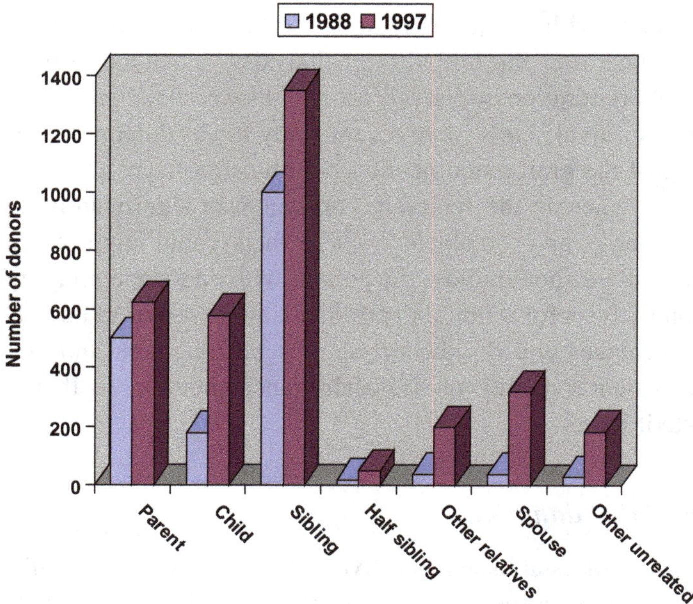

Figure 2: Relationship of live kidney donors to recipients in 1988 versus 1997 showing the increase in distant relatives and unrelated donors in the US.[42]

acceptable by using a simplified method with which the physician takes responsibility for the emotional relationship between donor and recipient, e.g. in the US where a signed declaration by both donor and recipient that they are spouses or partners is required. There are surgeons against spousal donation advising that since 30–40% of marriages end in divorce there is no guarantee of a long-lasting loving relationship as a motive for such donation.[66]

Friends have been accepted reluctantly as potential donors, despite the fact that they might feel less pressure to donate compared to a family member, although such practice has never been restricted.

Donation by strangers

In the past, the majority of transplant centres disapproved living donation between strangers (non-directed donation), expressing doubts about: (a) their motivation and commitment to donation; (b) their understanding of the potential risks and (c) their psychological stability.[67] Yet in recent surveys in the US, there is strong medical and public support for the acceptance of strangers as donors. Studies have found no regrets or psychological implications following non-directed donation.[68] Such donors may also benefit from their act with increased self-esteem and may experience even greater satisfaction without being coerced by any sense of obligation.

Researchers have proposed that in non-directed donation, the donor and recipient should remain anonymous to each other and probably meet only after the transplant, if they both agree.[69] It has been suggested that true altruists do not need the name of those they help.[70] In case anonymity is not respected there is a risk of future financial requests from the donor. Yet, we should acknowledge that the donor might want to see the results of their good deed, and the recipient might want to express their gratitude to the donor.

In 1996, a German professor of surgery and head of a transplant centre, Dr Jochem Hoyer, voluntarily donated a kidney to an unknown recipient chosen from the Munich waiting list. This has led to proposals, in Germany, of a registry for non-directed donors.[71] It seems unethical to allow potential donors to specify particular characteristics of the recipient (e.g. age or race) although some surgeons[72] have suggested that if people were allowed to donate to someone they feel connected to, the number of donated kidneys would rise. Finally, there are individuals that doubt that anyone would consider non-directed donation without any substantial reward.[73]

Commercialization of organ donation

Perhaps the hottest debate in live-donor transplantation nowadays is in regard to the potential financial rewards for the donor. In the UK, the Act of Parliament in 1990 made the sale of organs illegal and stipulated that proof of a relationship between donor and recipient must be genetically established before transplantation. This Act was produced after a General Medical Council's enquiry into a case of a British physician's involvement in transplants involving Turkish peasants.[65] As we mentioned earlier, in the UK the law requires that a renal transplant in which donor and recipient are not blood related relatives (including spouses) must be approved by the ULTRA, whose chairman is appointed by the Secretary of State for Health.[74] In the US, the transplant team is responsible for determining and assessing the motive of the donor, and the sale of organs is illegal. Yet the shortage of cadaveric organs has led to a worldwide black market for living-donor organs, with patients who possess the necessary means travelling to distant locations in order to purchase a kidney for transplantation.

On one hand we consider the purchase of organs as a hideous act (deontologial ethical approach), yet on the other we are obliged to consider ways to increase the live-donor pool (utilitarian ethical approach). For example, in Bombay, India, the price for a woman's kidney is alleged to be $1,000; in Manila, the Philippines, a man's kidney is said to be worth $2,000; and in urban Latin America a kidney can be sold for more than $10,000 with additional payments to the brokers in all the previous cases.[75] While Americans are purchasing kidneys from strangers in China, Peru and the Philippines, the current federal law does not prevent these patients from returning to the US for post-transplantation care.[76,77] Furthermore, there are also allegations that affluent patients from other countries have paid at least $200,000 to undergo transplantation at US centres, as part of a package pre-arranged outside the US by international brokers, including compensation for unrelated donors.[75]

Some of the arguments and counterarguments related to the commercialization of organ donation are as follows:

(a) It is unethical to sell your body or your organs, since the importance of life is paramount and every human being is special. Organs cannot be regarded as commodities for sale. For the same reasons that we cannot accept prostitution and child trading, we cannot endorse commerce of human organs. Some might argue that in a free society, the individual is entitled to do anything they want, including selling their organs, as long as they are not restricting the liberty of their fellow citizens.
(b) A poor donor is compelled by their financial status to donate, thus making the action non-voluntary. Yet, on the contrary, the donor may

be choosing the best from a list of bad options, since it carries significantly less risk than working, for example, under harsh and dangerous conditions, as well as offering them the pleasure of contributing to the well-being of the recipient. Although the recipient may be taking advantage of the donor's difficult economic situation, this will not improve by refusing donation.

(c) Paid donors are, in their majority, poor and less educated, thus possibly unable to understand the risks involved. But someone could easily argue that it is the physician's duty to explain the whole procedure as simply and clearly as possible, as well as to clarify every question raised by the potential donor.

(d) Another argument against commercialization of donation is that the rich will eventually have access to organs while the poor will not. However, it is also a fact of life that since private health care exists, the rich are able to buy better conditions of care than the poor.

(e) The sale of organs may also cause exploitation of donors and recipients by unscrupulous middlemen and surgeons. Yet, such practice may increase even more in an illegal uncontrolled environment resulting in the provision of inferior medical care. The financial exploitation of donors could be avoided if donation was supervised and controlled by a national agency which would allocate organs nationally according to best match and clinical need criteria as well as maintain the anonymity of the donor-recipient relationship.[78] In such setting, safety for the donor and the recipient would be guaranteed with better pre-, intra- and postoperative care for them.[79] However, if such a policy is applied on a larger scale it may lead to differences in financial compensation between transplant centres and even countries resulting in 'donation tourism' from poor to wealthy areas of the world.[79] Other researchers have also proposed a closely regulated and supervised market of organs, claiming that we do not regard this as any the less a caring profession because doctors are paid.[80] Since the long-term cost of renal transplantation is less compared to the patient on dialysis, the government or medical insurance organizations would save money. It has also been proposed[42] that wealthier patients could make financial contributions to a general and independent fund that would pay the potential donors, thus reducing the cost for the government even more. The initial selection and screening of the potential donor could be performed by an independent physician and then the transplant centre could have the right to reject them, after consulting a specialist on medical ethics. The paid donor would not be able to select a specific recipient. Others fear that rewarding donors will potentially lead to an increase in the cost of transplantation since those who now donate their kidneys altruistically might ask to be compensated.[81]

(f) Another argument against commercial donation is that the poor donor may be unable to handle their money well (compare with cases of lottery winners[42]) thus making in the long-term no difference to their poverty. The possibility of misuse of the money paid for donation, although difficult to predict, could not justify overriding the donor's decision.

(g) Transplantation has always relied to the altruism of donors and paid donation may lead to the disappearance of altruistic donation since it is possible that eventually all donors will request to be paid.

(h) Even if we manage to regulate the sale of organs, there is always the fear that some people will take it to the extreme; for example, the stories of Brazilian children, kidnapped and killed for their organs, as well as stories of people being drugged and kidnapped, awaking in an alley with a flank incision and a kidney missing.

(i) Others claim that living donation involves a 'highly artificial enforced altruism' according to which everyone is paid, including the transplant team, the transplant co-ordinator as well as the recipient who gains an important benefit and only the donor is required to be altruistic.[80] However, we have to acknowledge that those involved professionally with the transplant procedure do not receive extra payment for every transplant they perform and eventually it is their job to perform it.

(j) We could consider the scenario of an impoverished father who has a daughter ill with leukaemia. If his daughter experiences renal failure he would want to donate her his kidney. It could be morally acceptable in the eyes of some researchers[82] to sell his kidney in order to earn money to pay for her treatment. However, the counterargument is that in such cases a well-organized National Health Service should be able to provide the necessary resources and financial assistance for them.

(k) Others[83] consider it an act of paternalism that the rich are free to engage in dangerous sports for pleasure and the poor denied the smaller risk of selling a kidney, which may even save another life and help them with their financial situation. It is true that if kidney sales are allowed rich people will have opportunities for medical care unavailable to the poor, but this is a reality in many areas of medical care around the world and by outlawing such sales the social inequities will not be corrected.[84]

Information about several types of commercial donation is already available, although centres involved in such a practice would be reluctant to report results. One study looks at recipients who purchased a kidney in an Arab country and had follow-up with nephrologists after returning home. The results demonstrate a higher perioperative (6.2%) and three-month mortality rate (12.3%), as well as an almost 12% lower one-year survival rate (81.5%), when compared to the figures of non-related renal transplantation performed in the Western countries.[85] In this study, although the graft survival rate was similar to that of live unrelated transplants done in other countries in the Middle East, there was higher incidence of serious infections including HIV and Hepatitis B.[86] Another report on commercial transplantation showed a high rate of serious complications for Palestinian children suffering from end-stage renal disease who were transplanted in Iraq.[87] In another more recent study concerning Tunisian patients who purchased a kidney in Iraq (mean cost $10,000), Egypt and Pakistan, there was a very high complication rate.[88] Although there is still an organ black market in India, since dialysis is very expensive and cadaveric donations very rare, we have an early example of a paid donation programme,[89] which was suspended after commercial donation was made illegal. In this programme, before it became illegal, after careful screening of the donors, where even 72% were rejected, a two-year graft survival similar for related and unrelated donors was achieved. Those rejected were compensated for their time and the eventual donors were offered free three-year medical care. In Iran, there has been a compensated, controlled unrelated living-donor transplantation programme since 1988, which resulted in the elimination of the renal transplant list by 1999.[90] In this programme, the government pays all hospital expenses as well as provides the donor with an award and health insurance, without involving any middlemen or agency. Such a programme in the Middle-Eastern countries, where strong cultural barriers exist against cadaveric donation and long-term dialysis is unavailable or very limited, could reduce the over 50,000 annual deaths due to end-stage renal disease.[91] In a recent survey in Hungary[92] 63.3% of those interviewed, who already had been donors in the past, were not in favour of selling and buying organs, but, interestingly, they stated that if they had end-stage renal failure they would have bought a kidney if one had been available. Finally, there is great concern that no matter how well regulated an 'organ market' is, dubious brokers would find a way to bypass the regulated system and use other means to obtain a better price for an organ with prospective 'buyers' bidding for the best, medically most suitable one.[93]

Donor rewards

Even if we reject commercialization of donation, the question remains: should donors have any rewards at all? Most would agree that donors should at least not suffer from their donation, thus certain reasonable rewards are allowed. Researchers[19] have discovered that recipients and potential recipients were unwilling to accept a kidney if this would inflict any financial burden on the donors. Thus, if such a donor develops later renal failure, it is suggested that he could be placed at the top of the cadaveric kidney waiting list. He should also be provided with medical insurance and reimbursed for any lost working hours or lost wages.[94] Who could provide such compensation? It is generally accepted that this should be done by some government authority such as the NHS.[33] In the UK there are sophisticated mechanisms in place to calculate the loss of working hours or loss of wages and to compensate the donors fairly.

In 2001, during the first session of the 107th US Congress, new legislation was considered for the promotion of organ donation. It included the presentation of commemorative medals to donors, the offer of tax credits, as well as the reimbursement of travel and other expenses incurred as a result of donation. Also, a 30-day paid medical leave for all federal and some state employees, who become donors, was established. Moreover, the American Society of Transplantation (AST) is encouraging transplantation centres to provide paid medical leave for employees who become donors since they risk loss of wages or loss of employment.[75] The University of Minnesota offered a small financial aid in its transplantation programme intended to minimize donor expenses created by the procedure.[95] Also in Pennsylvania the state proposed a plan to offer $300 to organ donors and their families to be used only for expenses such as food, housing and transportation.[96]

The idea of non-cash rewards for donors might preserve the concept of altruism. The Red Cross gives, for example, T-shirts, food and drinks to those who donate blood but would not give their cash equivalent. The foundations of our society, life and liberty are values that should not have a monetary value. Thus, being awarded a medal or a certificate by the state for their generous action could be enough. This could happen in official ceremonies, thus gaining publicity through the media, which could further promote donation. The obligation of medical follow-up and the possibility of free health insurance is also a considerable reward for donors, expressing society's gratitude for such altruistic acts. The obligation of medical follow-up is also necessary in order to determine possible long-term risks for the sake of future donors and even if they are proven not to be in such a risk, their medical problems will be recognized and treated earlier. In a study in France,[97] two-thirds of the centres performed annual lifetime reviews for the donor, whereas the rest examined them once or twice before referring them to their personal physician for annual check-up (blood-pressure measurement, serum creatinine and screening for proteinuria).

Surrogate consent

The statement of the Live Organ Donor Consensus Group (LODCG) in 2000, that the donor should be competent to consent, rejects the idea of surrogates (patient's family) to consent to organ retrieval from an incompetent adult, although such examples appear occasionally[98] and have even been allowed.[99] In 1998, in Ohio, a judge ruled that a kidney could be removed from a patient in coma and given to his brother; since the patient's condition was irreversible, he could still live with one kidney and there was evidence that he had expressed the will to become an organ donor.[100] The family's decision to donate the kidney of a patient who lacks decision-making capacity is obviously not to the patient's benefit since they will probably never regain consciousness to realize the action. How is it then possible to justify such an action? First of all, when family members have proven that they are expressing the patient's will, his autonomy is respected. The adult in coma has a history of life choices, values and priorities that can help his family decide. A legal analysis argues that surrogates have to consider also the best interests of the family as a whole when making such decisions.[101]

A UCLA Medical Centre Ethics Committee[99] has proposed several principles for surrogate consent: (a) the family members should be able to prove that their decision is based on the patient's will; (b) surrogates should have no benefit from the donation except the satisfaction of their altruistic act; (c) the procedure should not affect the clinical course of the donor; (d) all the parties involved in the transplant procedure as well as those involved with the donor's care must believe that the donation is ethical and (e) the consent should be evaluated by an independent multidisciplinary body, such as an ethics committee, on a case-by-case basis.

Surrogate consent should be limited to patients with the least possibility of recovery and those who will die following withdrawal of life support. Such patients could be those in a permanent vegetative state (PVS). When the vegetative state lasts more than one month in cases with no injury, over three months in cases after non-traumatic injury and over 12 months in cases of traumatic injury, it is considered as permanent and their median survival is approximately two to five years.[102] Yet, are we able to determine whether a vegetative state is truly permanent? We can consider as an example the recent report of a person who recovered partially and started responding to questions after 19 years in coma.[103] That is why the surrogate should base their decision on what the patient would have chosen, regarding donation, if competent. Some[103] fear that allowing surrogates to donate non-vital organs (e.g. kidneys) of terminally-ill patients may undermine public trust in transplant programmes and expand donation to other patient groups, such as Alzheimer patients. Thus, they suggest that living-organ donation should be limited only to PVS patients.

Paired-exchange programmes

Another possible way to increase the live-donor pool is the paired-exchange programmes first suggested in 1986.[104] In such a programme pairs of potential donors who are incompatible with their recipients donate eventually to each other's recipient. Through an exchange arrangement between two donor-recipient pairs, donor A provides a kidney to (ABO-compatible) recipient D and donor C provides a kidney to (ABO-compatible) recipient B (Fig. 3).[105] Additionally, instead of direct exchange between pairs, donations could be made through an exchange donor pool. Such a programme was developed in Korea in 1991, resulting in a significant 7.3% increase of live-donor transplants.[106] The reasons for participating in the paired-exchange process were ABO incompatibility (75.5%), poor HLA-match (13.6%) and positive lymphocyte crossmatch (10.9%). The US also have experience with 'kidney swapping'.[107] In Europe paired-exchange transplantations have been attempted only in Switzerland, Romania and the Netherlands.

The consensus statement in 2000[32] stated that the meeting of the donor-recipient pairs remains at their, as well as at the transplant centre's, discretion. A survey[108] performed among potential pairs participating in

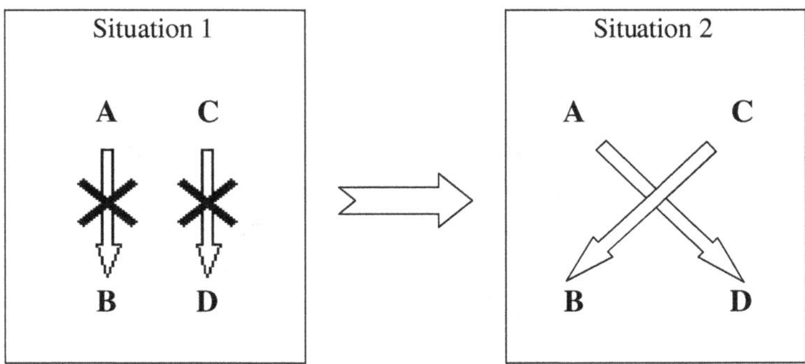

Figure 3: Paired-exchange programme. Live-donor kidney transplantation cannot happen for reasons such as blood group incompatibility between otherwise suitable donor and recipient (donor A to recipient B). The same can potentially stand for another pair of donor and recipient (donor C and recipient D). However if donor A gives a kidney to recipient D and donor C to recipient B, both transplantations are possible. An exchange of kidneys between two donor-recipient pairs.

an exchange programme concluded that all preferred anonymity, instead of becoming emotionally involved with others with similar health problems, avoiding psychological pressure that might result from acquaintance. Others[105] have suggested that strict confidentiality should be maintained for each donor-recipient pair because there is a possibility of frustration, anger or resentment between the two pairs, in case one recipient does not have such a good outcome as the other. It also suggested that both procedures should be performed simultaneously in order to avoid the possibility of one donor refusing after the other donor nephrectomy procedure had already been performed. It has also been suggested that in pair-exchange programmes, the psychological pressure on the donor may be greater since they are asked to give a kidney to a stranger rather than a loved one. Nonetheless, potential donors can understand that their donation will benefit indirectly their loved ones. Another ethical aspect of such a programme is the possibility of coercion since a reluctant donor cannot use an excuse such as ABO incompatibility for not donating. Thus, psychological evaluation should be more meticulous to ensure that the donor is acting voluntarily. Yet, with the advances in immunosuppression and plasma-exchange techniques, such programmes may be unnecessary, since ABO- and HLA-crossmatch incompatible transplants may be possible.

Minor donors

Another important issue under debate is whether minors, children younger than 18 years old, should be allowed to donate. The majority of kidneys transplanted to children come from their parents. However, this is not always possible for medical or other reasons. Should minors be allowed to donate to their siblings? From whom is consent required and who should decide about such a transplant? What should the minimum age be for donation?

There are some serious concerns about children donors. First of all, a child may be unable to balance and comprehend the risks and benefits of the procedure, thus may not be able to provide valid informed consent. Also, children may feel coerced by parents to donate and have no choice in the matter, risking parental love and support in that they go against their parents' wishes. Furthermore, parents may face a conflict of interests when a healthy child is considering donation in order to help their ill child.[109] Finally, there are some extra risks, although limited, to the child with one remaining kidney, such as risk for trauma, neoplasm and infection that can alter their physical activity, and possibly their choice of a career, for example limiting their ability in careers such as athletics, the military, etc.[110] Preadolescent and adolescent years are very important for the emotional, physical and intellectual development of a minor, thus there should be good justification to interrupt this process with an operation that is not medically required. We have to take into account issues of postoperative convalescence and disruption of school, activities, play, etc., which are essential in the daily life of a child at a formative age.

There is a view that we must consider older and younger children separately.[109] According to this view, formal operational thought has usually become well established in a child at about the age of 14, with adolescents being as competent as adults to make decisions regarding their health. In 1994, the Council on Ethical and Judicial Affairs of the American Medical Association considered adolescents of 14 years old and above, as mature enough to make decisions about their medical care, but this capacity should be evaluated in each individual case. Thus, several states in the US grant such 'mature minors' the right to provide consent to medical treatment intended for their benefit.[109] Before accepting an adolescent's consent, competence should be evaluated by a skilled mental health professional after consultation with the parents, who should also agree to donation. In addition, the child's competence should also be confirmed by courts as recommended by the Council on Ethical and Judicial Affairs of the American Medical Association. Data from this Council suggest that parental influence on children's decisions decreases as the children get older. In a previous study,[111] comprising young donors (16–20 years old), the vast majority appeared to be under no family pressure to donate and, one year after donating, most of them had not regretted it. The aforementioned Council also recommended that health professionals and the courts should also confirm that the adolescent is acting voluntarily. As Aaron Spital postulated 'although court involvement seems reasonable, it may be that a determination of competency and voluntarism can be achieved less traumatically, more efficiently, and at least as accurately by qualified health professionals alone'.[109]

Regarding the risk of nephrectomy in childhood, a large study[112] concluded that renal function is maintained for up to 50 years after unilateral nephrectomy in childhood. Thus, it may be too restrictive for transplant centres to accept kidney donors only over 18 years old. As Hamburger and Crosnier pointed out, it is really difficult to accept an age limit beneath which a minor is rejected as a donor since consideration should depend on the psychological maturity rather than the chronologic age of the child.[113] As a result, some states in the US have started to legally accept the consent of minors over 14 years old for organ and tissue donation, e.g. in Alabama minors can consent for bone marrow donation and in Michigan they can be kidney donors to immediate family members with court approval.[109]

However, it is very difficult to accept 'immature' minors (under 14 years old) as donors, since they are unable to make sound decisions regarding their own health and their choices are influenced greatly by their parents. On the other hand, one could argue that this approach is very restrictive and under rare circumstances even young minors should be allowed to donate.[109] Considering this approach, we must acknowledge that legislation accepts an incompetent individual as a potential donor only if donation is in the individual's best interests and they benefit from it. Similar psychological benefits for young children have been used by courts as justifications for approving donations by minors, whereas these benefits have actually been documented in a 7-year-old donor.[114] Some of the benefits for a young child after donation could be: (a) avoiding trauma caused by the death of a very close relative e.g. a sibling; (b) avoiding future emotions of guilt for not donating; (c) increased self-esteem from donation; (d) maintaining the integrity of the family in which they live.[109] However, we should always keep in mind that we can only speculate rather than be certain about the psychological benefits to the child-donor. That is the reason why the Council on Ethical and Judicial Affairs of the American Medical Association has proposed that organ donation from an 'immature' minor potential donor should only be permitted if parents and courts agree 'that donation could provide a "clear benefit" to the donor'.[115] It is also recommended that the minor is evaluated by a child psychiatrist

Table 5: Attitudes towards the use of minors as live kidney donors among 99 responding US transplant centres in 1989[117] and among 117 responding US transplant centres in 1997.[109]

	Would consider		Would not consider		Did not answer	
Donor source	1989	1997	1989	1997	1989	1997
Monozygotic twin	64%	42%	32%	56%	4%	2%
Non-twin sibling	43%	25%	53%	75%	4%	—

or psychologist and a guardian is appointed on the minor's behalf to ensure the protection of the child's interests.[116] This procedure would require stringent safeguards such as: (a) the child is the only available organ source; (b) the transplant procedure has a very high possibility of success; (c) the recipient will benefit from the transplant; (d) the recipient is a close family member; (e) the potential donor will likely benefit from the procedure; (f) the risk of donation is extremely small; (g) the child freely agrees to the procedure, requiring the child to be old enough for that decision, probably over 7 years old.[109] Although these concepts reject a definite ban on donation by young children, they limit greatly the number of minors who can be considered as potential donors.

Surveys[109] that have been performed in transplant centres in the US have demonstrated that the acceptance of children as live donors is decreasing (Table 5) compared to the attitudes described in a previous study[117] while there is great controversy regarding the issue of the donor's acceptable age (Fig. 4).[109] Finally, in the most recent of those studies,[109] the centres that would sometimes accept minors as donors required consent from: parents (88%), the minor donor (75%), a court (69%) and an appointed guardian (50%).

Conclusion

The many ethical issues regarding live-donor organ transplantation have been under intense debate, with much controversy and a range of ideas and practices existing between countries, transplant centres and physicians.

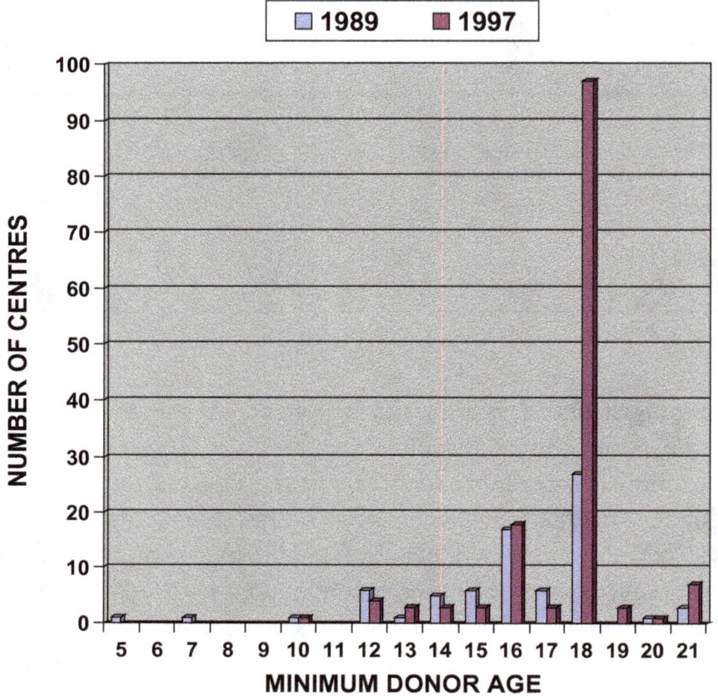

Figure 4: Minimum donor age acceptable by 74 responding US transplant centres in 1989[117] and by 143 responding US transplant centres in 1997.[109]

Cultural, socioeconomic and demographic factors make those issues even more complicated. However, we believe that, following an open and honest debate involving all the interested parties, an agreement on certain generally accepted principles can be achieved. Such an agreement will safeguard the potential donors, recipients and their families and can only boost the future of live-donor transplantation.

References

1. Dossetor JB, Daar AS. Ethics in transplantation: allotransplantation and xenotransplantation. In *Kidney Transplantation. Principles and Practice*. 5th edn. Ed: P Morris. Philadelphia: WB Saunders Company. 2001, pp 732–44.

2. Cecka JM. The UNOS renal transplant registry. *Clin. Transpl.* 2002: 1–20.
3. Rothenberg LS. Ethical and legal issues in kidney transplantation. In *Handbook of Kidney Transplantation*. Ed: GM Danovitch. Philadelphia: Lippincott Williams & Wilkins. 2001, pp 380–93.
4. Papalois V, Vlachos K, Barlas A, Zarka ZA, El-Tayar A, Hakim NS. Ethical issues in non-heart-beating donation. *Bull. Med. Ethics* 2004;202: 13–20.
5. Gohh RY, Morrissey PE, Madras PN, Monaco AP. Controversies in organ donation: the altruistic living donor. *Nephrol. Dial. Transplant* 2001;16(3): 619–21.
6. Kasiske BL, Bia MJ. The evaluation and selection of living kidney donors. *Am. J. Kidney Dis.* 1995;26(2):387–98.
7. Johnson EM, Remucal MJ, Gillingham KJ, Dahms RA, Najarian JS, Matas AJ. Complications and risks of living-donor nephrectomy. *Transplantation* 1997;64(8):1124–8.
8. Johnson EM, Anderson JK, Jacobs C, Suh G, Humar A, Suhr BD, *et al.* Long-term follow-up of living kidney donors: quality of life after donation. *Transplantation* 1999;67(5):717–21.
9. Corley MC, Elswick RK, Sargeant CC, Scott S. Attitude, self-image, and quality of life of living kidney donors. *Nephrol. Nurs. J.* 2000;27(1):43–50; discussion 51–2.
10. de Graaf Olson W, Bogetti-Dumlao A. Living donors' perception of their quality of health after donation. *Prog. Transplant* 2001;11(2):108–15.
11. Ramcharan T, Matas AJ. Long-term (20–37 years) follow-up of living kidney donors. *Am. J. Transplant* 2002;2(10):959–64.
12. Ozcurumez G, Tanriverdi N, Colak T, Emiroglu R, Zileli L, Haberal M. The psychosocial impact of renal transplantation on living related donors and recipients: preliminary report. *Transplant Proc.* 2004;36(1):114–16.
13. Bay WH, Hebert LA. The living donor in kidney transplantation. *Ann. Intern. Med.* 1987;106(5):719–27.
14. Najarian JS, Chavers BM, McHugh LE, Matas AJ. Twenty years or more of follow-up of living kidney donors. *Lancet* 1992;340(8823):807–10.
15. Goldfarb DA, Matin SF, Braun WE, Schreiber MJ, Mastroianni B, Papajcik D, *et al.* Renal outcome 25 years after donor nephrectomy. *J. Urol.* 2001;166(6):2043–7.

16. Narkun-Burgess DM, Nolan CR, Norman JE, Page WF, Miller PL, Meyer TW. Forty-five year follow-up after uninephrectomy. *Kidney Int.* 1993;43(5): 1110–15.
17. Hakim N, Zarka ZA, El-Tayar A, Mustafa N, Papalois V. A fast and safe living-donor nephrectomy technique. *Transplant Proc.* 2003;35(7):2555–6.
18. Ratner LE, Kavoussi LR, Schulam PG, Bender JS, Magnuson TH, Montgomery R. Comparison of laparoscopic live-donor nephrectomy versus the standard open approach. *Transplant Proc.* 1997;29(1–2):138–9.
19. Pradel FG, Mullins CD, Bartlett ST. Exploring donors' and recipients' attitudes about living-donor kidney transplantation. *Prog. Transplant* 2003;13(3): 203–10.
20. Chiu AW, Azadzoi KM, Hatzichristou DG, Siroky MB, Krane RJ, Babayan RK. Effects of intra-abdominal pressure on renal tissue perfusion during laparoscopy. *J. Endourol.* 1994;8(2):99–103.
21. Chiu AW, Chang LS, Birkett DH, Babayan RK. The impact of pneumoperitoneum, pneumoretroperitoneum and gasless laparoscopy on the systemic and renal hemodynamics. *J. Am. Coll. Surg.* 1995;181(5):397–406.
22. Spital A. Life insurance for kidney donors — an update. *Transplantation* 1988;45(4):819–20.
23. Lennerling A, Forsberg A, Meyer K, Nyberg G. Motives for becoming a living kidney donor. *Nephrol. Dial. Transplant* 2004;19(6):1600–5.
24. Lennerling A, Forsberg A, Nyberg G. Becoming a living kidney donor. *Transplantation* 2003;76(8):1243–7.
25. Schover LR, Streem SB, Boparai N, Duriak K, Novick AC. The psychosocial impact of donating a kidney: long-term follow-up from a urology-based center. *J. Urol.* 1997;157(5):1596–601.
26. Isotani S, Fujisawa M, Ichikawa Y, Ishimura T, Matsumoto O, Hamami G, *et al.* Quality of life of living kidney donors: the short-form 36-item health questionnaire survey. *Urology* 2002;60(4):588–92; discussion 592.
27. Schostak M, Wloch H, Muller M, Schrader M, Offermann G, Miller K. Optimizing open live-donor nephrectomy — long-term donor outcome. *Clin. Transplant* 2004;18(3):301–5.
28. Franklin PM, Crombie AK. Live related renal transplantation: psychological, social, and cultural issues. *Transplantation* 2003;76(8):1247–52.
29. Griva K, Ziegelmann JP, Thompson D, Jayasena D, Davenport A, Harrison M, *et al.* Quality of life and emotional responses in cadaver and living

related renal transplant recipients. *Nephrol. Dial. Transplant* 2002;17(12): 2204–11.

30. Baines LS, Beattie TJ, Murphy AV, Jindal RM. Relationship between donors and pediatric recipients of kidney transplants: a psychosocial study. *Transplant Proc.* 2001;33(1–2):1897–9.
31. Gordon EJ. 'They don't have to suffer for me': why dialysis patients refuse offers of living-donor kidneys. *Med. Anthropol. Q.* 2001;15(2):245–67.
32. Abecassis M, Adams M, Adams P, Arnold RM, Atkins CR, Barr ML, *et al.* Consensus statement on the live-organ donor. *JAMA* 2000;284(22):2919–26.
33. Steiner RW, Gert B. Ethical selection of living kidney donors. *Am. J. Kidney Dis.* 2000;36(4):677–86.
34. Boulware LE, Ratner LE, Sosa JA, Tu AH, Nagula S, Simpkins CE, *et al.* The general public's concerns about clinical risk in live kidney donation. *Am. J. Transplant* 2002;2(2):186–93.
35. Burroughs TE, Waterman AD, Hong BA. One organ donation, three perspectives: experiences of donors, recipients, and third parties with living kidney donation. *Prog. Transplant* 2003;13(2):142–50.
36. Smith GC, Trauer T, Kerr PG, Chadban SJ. Prospective psychosocial monitoring of living kidney donors using the SF-36 health survey. *Transplantation* 2003;76(5):807–9.
37. Eggeling C. The psychosocial implications of live-related kidney donation. *Edtna Erca J.* 1999;25(3):19–22.
38. Spital A. Ethical issues in living-organ donation: donor autonomy and beyond. *Am. J. Kidney Dis.* 2001;38(1):189–95.
39. Ross LF. Donating a second kidney: a tale of family and ethics. *Semin. Dial.* 2000;13(3):201–3.
40. Crouch RA, Elliott C. Moral agency and the family: the case of living related organ transplantation. *Camb. Q. Healthc. Ethics* 1999;8(3):275–87.
41. Russell S, Jacob RG. Living related organ donation: the donor's dilemma. *Patient Educ. Couns.* 1993;21(1–2):89–99.
42. Hou S. Expanding the kidney donor pool: ethical and medical considerations. *Kidney Int.* 2000;58(4):1820–36.
43. Spital A. The ethics of unconventional living organ donation. *Clin. Transplant* 1991;5(4):322–6.
44. Cicciarelli J, Iwaki Y, Mendez R. The influence of donor age on kidney graft survival in the 1990s. *Clin. Transpl.* 1999:335–40.

45. Prommool S, Jhangri GS, Cockfield SM, Halloran PF. Time dependency of factors affecting renal allograft survival. *J. Am. Soc. Nephrol.* 2000;11(3): 565–73.
46. Sakellariou G, Daniilidis M, Alexopoulos E, Karagiannis A, Papadimitriou M. Does the donor age influence graft survival in renal transplantation? *Transplant Proc.* 1987;19(1 Pt 3):2071–3.
47. Kwon OJ, Lee HG, Kwak JY. The impact of donor and recipient age on the outcome of kidney transplantation. *Transplant Proc.* 2004;36(7):2043–5.
48. Bleyer AJ, Burkart JM, Russell GB, Adams PL. Dialysis modality and delayed graft function after cadaveric renal transplantation. *J. Am. Soc. Nephrol.* 1999;10(1):154–9.
49. Cosio FG, Alamir A, Yim S, Pesavento TE, Falkenhain ME, Henry ML, *et al.* Patient survival after renal transplantation: I. The impact of dialysis pre-transplant. *Kidney Int.* 1998;53(3):767–72.
50. Mange KC, Joffe MM, Feldman HI. Effect of the use or non-use of long-term dialysis on the subsequent survival of renal transplants from living donors. *N. Engl. J. Med.* 2001;344(10):726–31.
51. Mange KC, Joffe MM, Feldman HI. Dialysis prior to living-donor kidney transplantation and rates of acute rejection. *Nephrol. Dial. Transplant* 2003;18(1):172–7.
52. Meier-Kriesche H, Port FK, Ojo AO, Leichtman AB, Rudich SM, Arndorfer JA, *et al.* Deleterious effect of waiting time on renal transplant outcome. *Transplant Proc.* 2001;33(1–2):1204–6.
53. Papalois VE, Moss A, Gillingham KJ, Sutherland DE, Matas AJ, Humar A. Pre-emptive transplants for patients with renal failure: an argument against waiting until dialysis. *Transplantation* 2000;70(4):625–31.
54. Kasiske BL, Snyder JJ, Matas AJ, Ellison MD, Gill JS, Kausz AT. Pre-emptive kidney transplantation: the advantage and the advantaged. *J. Am. Soc. Nephrol.* 2002;13(5):1358–64.
55. Goldfarb-Rumyantzev A, Hurdle JF, Scandling J, Wang Z, Baird B, Barenbaum L, *et al.* Duration of end-stage renal disease and kidney transplant outcome. *Nephrol. Dial. Transplant* 2005;20(1):167–75.
56. Kikuchi K, Narumi Y, Hama K, Iwamoto H, Uchiyama M, Kozaki K, *et al.* Kidney transplantation from spousal donors. *Transplant Proc.* 2000;32(7): 1817–18.

57. Tang S, Lui SL, Lo CY, Lo WK, Cheng IK, Lai KN, *et al.* Spousal renal donor transplantation in Chinese subjects: a ten-year experience from a single centre. *Nephrol. Dial. Transplant* 2004;19(1):203–6.
58. Bruzzone P, Pretagostini R, Rossi M, Berloco PB. Ethical considerations on kidney transplantation from living donors. *Ann. Transplant* 2004;9(2):46–7.
59. Spital A. Do US transplant centres encourage emotionally related kidney donation? *Transplantation* 1996;61(3):374–7.
60. Terasaki PI, Cecka JM, Gjertson DW, Cho YW. Spousal and other living renal donor transplants. *Clin. Transpl.* 1997:269–84.
61. Watanabe T, Hiraga S. Influence on family psychodynamics on spousal kidney transplantation. *Transplant Proc.* 2002;34(4):1145–7.
62. Thiel G. Emotionally related living kidney donation: pro and contra. *Nephrol. Dial. Transplant* 1997;12(9):1820–4.
63. Soulillou JP. Kidney transplantation from spousal donors. *N. Engl. J. Med.* 1995;333(6):379–80.
64. Mathieson PW, Jolliffe D, Jolliffe R, Dudley CR, Hamilton K, Lear PA. The spouse as a kidney donor: ethically sound? *Nephrol. Dial. Transplant* 1999;14(1):46–8.
65. Choudhry S, Daar AS, Radcliffe Richards J, Guttmann RD, Hoffenberg R, Lock M, *et al.* Unrelated living organ donation: ULTRA needs to go. *J. Med. Ethics* 2003;29(3):169–70.
66. Isoniemi H. Living kidney donation; a surgeon's opinion. *Nephrol. Dial. Transplant* 1997;12(9):1828–9.
67. Fellner CH, Schwartz SH. Altruism in disrepute. Medical versus public attitudes toward the living-organ donor. *N. Engl. J. Med.* 1971;284(11):582–5.
68. Sadler HH, Davison L, Carroll C, Kountz SL. The living, genetically unrelated, kidney donor. *Semin. Psychiatry* 1971;3(1):86–101.
69. Matas AJ, Garvey CA, Jacobs CL, Kahn JP. Non-directed donation of kidneys from living donors. *N. Engl. J. Med.* 2000;343(6):433–6.
70. Kaplan BS, Polise K. In defense of altruistic kidney donation by strangers. *Pediatr. Nephrol.* 2000;14(6):518–22.
71. Rittner CK, Besold A, Wandel E. A proposal for an anonymous living-organ donation in Germany. *Leg. Med.* (Tokyo) 2003;5(Suppl 1):S68–71.
72. Spital A. Must kidney donation by living strangers be non-directed? *Transplantation* 2001;72(5):966.

73. Broyer M, Affleck J. In defense of altruistic kidney donation by strangers: a commentary. *Pediatr. Nephrol.* 2000;14(6):523–4.
74. http://www.doh.gov.uk/ultra.htm. In: Department of Health United Kingdom, Department of Health, Crown Copyright 1998.
75. Delmonico FL, Arnold R, Scheper-Hughes N, Siminoff LA, Kahn J, Youngner SJ. Ethical incentives — not payment — for organ donation. *N. Engl. J. Med.* 2002;346(25):2002–5.
76. Scheper-Hughes N. The global traffic in human organs. *Curr. Anthropol.* 2000;41(2):191–224.
77. Smith CS. On death row, China's source of transplants. *NY Times* (Print) 2001:A1, A10.
78. Mansell MA. The ethics of rewarded kidney donation. *BJU Int.* 2004;93(9):1171–2.
79. Schlitt HJ. Paid non-related living-organ donation: Horn of Plenty or Pandora's box? *Lancet* 2002;359(9310):906–7.
80. Harris J. In praise of unprincipled ethics. *J. Med. Ethics* 2003;29(5): 303–6.
81. Abouna GM. Negative impact of trading in human organs on the development of transplantation in the Middle East. *Transplant Proc.* 1993;25(3): 2310–13.
82. Levine DZ. Kidney vending: 'Yes!' or 'No!' *Am. J. Kidney Dis.* 2000;35(5): 1002–18.
83. Radcliffe-Richards J, Daar AS, Guttmann RD, Hoffenberg R, Kennedy I, Lock M, *et al.* The case for allowing kidney sales. International Forum for Transplant Ethics. *Lancet* 1998;351(9120):1950–2.
84. Grazi RV, Wolowelsky JB. Nonaltruistic kidney donations in contemporary Jewish law and ethics. *Transplantation* 2003;75(2):250–2.
85. Salahudeen AK, Woods HF, Pingle A, Nur-El-Huda Suleyman M, Shakuntala K, Nandakumar M, *et al.* High mortality among recipients of bought living unrelated donor kidneys. *Lancet* 1990;336(8717):725–8.
86. The Living Non-Related Renal Transplant Study Group. Commercially motivated renal transplantation: results in 540 patients transplanted in India. *Clin. Transplant* 1997;11(6):536–44.
87. Frishberg Y, Feinstein S, Drukker A. Living unrelated (commercial) renal transplantation in children. *J. Am. Soc. Nephrol.* 1998;9(6):1100–3.

88. Ben Hamida F, Ben Abdallah T, Goucha R, Hedri H, Helal I, Karoui C, *et al.* Outcome of living unrelated (commercial) renal transplantation: report of 20 cases. *Transplant Proc.* 2001;33(5):2660–1.
89. Thiagarajan CM, Reddy KC, Shunmugasundaram D, Jayachandran R, Nayar P, Thomas S, *et al.* The practice of unconventional renal transplantation (UCRT) at a single centre in India. *Transplant Proc.* 1990;22(3):912–14.
90. Ghods AJ. Changing ethics in renal transplantation: presentation of Iran model. *Transplant Proc.* 2004;36(1):11–13.
91. Ghods AJ. Should we have live unrelated donor renal transplantation in MESOT countries? *Transplant Proc.* 2003;35(7):2542–4.
92. Toronyi E, Alfoldy F, Jaray J, Remport A, Mathe Z, Szabo J, *et al.* Attitudes of donors towards organ transplantation in living related kidney transplantations. *Transpl. Int.* 1998;11(Suppl 1):S481–3.
93. Rothman DJ. Ethical and social consequences of selling a kidney. *JAMA* 2002;288(13):1640–1.
94. Wolters HH, Heidenreich S, Senninger N. Living-donor kidney transplantation: chance for the recipient — financial risk for the donor? *Transplant Proc.* 2003;35(6):2091–2.
95. Gridelli B, Remuzzi G. Strategies for making more organs available for transplantation. *N. Engl. J. Med.* 2000;343(6):404–10.
96. Yen H. PA plans financial aid for organ donors. *Philadelphia Inquirer* 2000 March 30;Sect. March 30, B03.
97. Gabolde M, Herve C, Moulin AM. Evaluation, selection, and follow-up of live kidney donors: a review of current practice in French renal transplant centres. *Nephrol. Dial. Transplant* 2001;16(10):2048–52.
98. Schlessinger S, Crook ED, Black R, Barber H. Ethical issues in transplantation: living related donation in the setting of severe neurological damage without brain death. *Am. J. Med. Sci.* 2002;324(4):232–6.
99. Brown-Saltzman K, Diamant A, Fineberg IC, Gritsch HA, Keane M, Korenman S, *et al.* Surrogate consent for living related organ donation. *JAMA* 2004;291(6):728–31.
100. Bramstedt KA. Surrogate consent for live-organ donation. *JAMA* 2004;291(17):2077–8; author reply 2078.
101. Morley MT. Proxy consent to organ donation by incompetents. *Yale Law J.* 2002;111(5):1215–49.

102. Ashwal S, Cranford R. Medical aspects of the persistent vegetative state — a correction. The Multi-Society Task Force on PVS. *N. Engl. J. Med.* 1995;333(2):130.
103. Wendler D, Emanuel E. Assessing the ethical and practical wisdom of surrogate consent for living-organ donation. *JAMA* 2004;291(6):732–5.
104. Rapaport FT. The case for a living emotionally related international kidney donor exchange registry. *Transplant Proc.* 1986;18(3 Suppl 2):5–9.
105. Ross LF, Rubin DT, Siegler M, Josephson MA, Thistlethwaite JR, Jr, Woodle ES. Ethics of a paired-kidney-exchange program. *N. Engl. J. Med.* 1997;336(24):1752–5.
106. Park K, Moon JI, Kim SI, Kim YS. Exchange donor program in kidney transplantation. *Transplantation* 1999;67(2):336–8.
107. McLellan F. US surgeons do first 'triple-swap' kidney transplantation. *Lancet* 2003;362(9382):456.
108. Kranenburg LW, Visak T, Weimar W, Zuidema W, de Klerk M, Hilhorst M, *et al.* Starting a crossover kidney transplantation program in the Netherlands: ethical and psychological considerations. *Transplantation* 2004;78(2): 194–7.
109. Spital A. Should children ever donate kidneys? Views of US transplant centres. *Transplantation* 1997;64(2):232–6.
110. Salvatierra O, Jr. Transplant physicians bear full responsibility for the consequences of kidney donation by a minor. *Am. J. Transplant* 2002;2(4): 297–8.
111. Bernstein DM, Simmons RG. The adolescent kidney donor: the right to give. *Am. J. Psychiatry* 1974;131(12):1338–43.
112. Baudoin P, Provoost AP, Molenaar JC. Renal function up to 50 years after unilateral nephrectomy in childhood. *Am. J. Kidney Dis.* 1993;21(6): 603–11.
113. Hamburger J, Crosnier J. Moral and ethical problems in transplantation. In *Human Transplantation.* Eds: F Rapaport F and J Daussert. New York: Grunn and Stratton. 1968.
114. Lewis M. Kidney donation by a 7-year-old identical twin child: psychological, legal, and ethical considerations. *J. Am. Acad. Child Psychiatry* 1974;13(2):221–45.
115. Council in Ethical and Judicial Affairs AMA. The use of minors as organ and tissue donors. *Code Med. Ethics Rep.* 1994;5:229.

116. Santiago-Delpin E. Additional guidelines on the use of minors as living kidney donors. *Am. J. Transplant* 2003;3(9):1182.
117. Spital A. Unconventional living kidney donors — attitudes and use among transplant centres. *Transplantation* 1989;48(2):243–8.

Chapter 2

Live Kidney Transplantation

Nicos Kessaris, Vassilios Papalois, Ruben Canelo and Nadey Hakim

Introduction

The first successful live kidney transplant was performed by Joseph Murray on 23 December 1954 at the Peter Bent Brigham Hospital in Boston.[1–3] The graft functioned immediately. The recipient survived for nine years, without immunosuppression, until the kidney failed due to recurrent glomerulonephritis. In the UK, the first successful renal transplant was performed by Michael Woodruff on 30 October 1960 at the Royal Infirmary of Edinburgh.[4] Since then there have been thousands of such transplants throughout the world.

With the increase in the number of patients on the cadaveric transplant waiting list and the reduction of cadaveric donors, the focus is on ways to expand the donor pool. Live transplantation is one vital way of accomplishing this. Table 1 shows the number of live transplants performed in the UK between 2001 and 2006. The observed increase in the number of live kidney transplants over this period has been attributed to improved surgical techniques, such as mini-open and laparoscopic nephrectomy, as well as to the appointment of specific coordinators dedicated to living donation.[5]

The increase in live-donor operations has also been observed in the USA. Since 2001, the number of live kidney donors in the USA has surpassed the number of cadaveric donors.[6–8] This trend has again been attributed to improved surgical techniques as well as to increased public awareness.[7,8]

Table 1: Number of live kidney transplants performed in the UK between 2001 and 2006.[9–13]

Period	Number of live transplants in UK	Percentage increase from previous year
2001–2002	372	N/A
2002–2003	376	1%
2003–2004	450	20%
2004–2005	475	6%
2005–2006	590	24%

As immunosuppression has improved with time, there has been a significant enhancement in graft outcome from live donors[14] as well as in recipient outcome. In a study from the US, the half-life of a live kidney graft increased from 12.7 to 21.6 years from 1988 to 1996.[14] This study also illustrated the advantage of longer graft survival from a live donor when compared with that from a cadaveric donor. Indeed the half-life of a cadaveric kidney graft only increased from 7.9 to 13.8 years during the same period.[14] This superior graft and recipient outcome improves further with pre-emptive transplantation.[8]

A live donor may be related or unrelated. Renal graft outcome from living unrelated donors have a similar three-year survival rate as grafts from living related donors despite having a worse match for HLA.[15] This is very important as spouses, as well as friends are significant sources of live kidney grafts.

Disadvantages of donation may be short term or long term.[16] These include a risk of 2% for a major complication[5,17] and a risk of 0.03% for death.[5,17,18] Therefore, optimal donor evaluation and informed consent is paramount.

The Donor

Donor evaluation

Potential donors are evaluated according to locally agreed, evidence-based protocols. In the UK, these are based on the standards and guidelines provided by the British Transplantation Society (BTS) and the Renal Association.[5] International guidelines have also been developed.[19]

Medical evaluation

Once a potential recipient is found to be fit for transplantation, evaluation of the potential donor can commence. This necessitates a preliminary medical assessment, either by a general practitioner, a live-donor coordinator or a nephrologist, where donors are screened for major contraindications to proceeding. It involves a brief history and examination followed by ABO and HLA typing as well as crossmatching. Recently, it has been possible to perform transplants between ABO incompatible patients. This is discussed in more detail below. This visit also allows information leaflets to be given to the potential donor about donation.

After this initial assessment a full medical evaluation is performed by a nephrologist. This involves taking a thorough medical history paying special emphasis on the past medical history as well as the psychosocial state (Table 2). It is followed by a general examination as well as a cardiorespiratory and abdominal examination (Table 2).

Table 2: Summary of history and examination of the potential donor.[5,20]

History

Age

Current medical problems

Past medical history including

- Cardiovascular disease (ischaemic heart disease, hypertension, stroke)
- Respiratory disease
- Gastrointestinal disease
- Renal disease (history or kidney stones, haematuria, infections and any treatments)
- Diabetes
- Infections
- Malignancy
- Neurological disease
- Thrombo-embolic disease

(*Continued*)

Table 2: (*Continued*)

Drug history including

- Antihypertensive medication
- Contraceptive pill

Family history including

- Cardiovascular disease
- Renal disease
- Diabetes

Psychosocial history

- Psychiatric disease
- Type of work
- Smoking
- Weight

Examination

General examination including

- Weight, height and Body Mass Index

Cardiovascular examination including

- Heart rate, blood pressure

Respiratory examination
Abdominal examination

Investigations

Provided no medical contraindications have been identified in the history or the examination, routine investigations are instigated. These are summarized in Table 3. The live-donor coordinator is vital in organizing and following up the investigations as well as guiding the donors throughout this process.

Surgical evaluation

Once the potential donor is investigated and found eligible for donation, he or she is seen in the clinic by the transplant surgeon. Here the donor is

Table 3: Routine investigations for potential live kidney donors based on the West London Renal and Transplant Centre Protocol, Hammersmith Hospital, Du Cane Road, London W12 0HS and the British Transplantation Society Guidelines.[5]

Type of investigation	Investigation
Haematology	• Full blood count • Clotting • Sickle cell test (where indicated) • Thrombophilia screen (where indicated)
Chemistry	• Renal profile • Liver function • Bone profile • Fasting serum glucose • Glucose tolerance test (if fasting glucose of 6–7 mmol/l)[21] • Lipid profile
Virology	• Hepatitis B, C • Cytomegalovirus • HIV I, II • Epstein-Barr Virus • Toxoplasma • Syphilis
Cardiology	• Chest X-ray • Electrocardiogram • Exercise stress test (where indicated) • Echocardiogram (where indicated)
Urinalysis	• Urine dipstick • Mid-stream urine for microscopy, culture and sensitivity
Renal imaging	• Renal/abdominal ultrasound scan
Renal function	• 24-hour urine collection for protein and creatinine clearance • EDTA or DTPA GFR measurement • DMSA scan
Angiography	• Magnetic Resonance or CT angiography to define vessel anatomy

evaluated in a similar way by history and examination. Then the procedure, as well as the risks associated with it, is explained to the donor. Time is given for answering any questions the donor may have.

Multidisciplinary evaluation

The week before donation a multidisciplinary meeting is carried out to review the donor's notes, results and imaging. People attending such a meeting include the live-donor coordinator, the transplant surgeon, the nephrologists but may also include a radiologist.

Assessment of renal function

Creatinine is a breakdown product of skeletal muscle. It is produced at a constant rate and mainly excreted by glomerular filtration. As serum creatinine does not start to rise until a substantial decline in GFR, it is not a very useful screening test for renal failure.[22]

Creatinine clearance can be estimated using a 24-hour urine collection. This may underestimate or overestimate GFR in patients with near normal or normal kidney function.[19]

GFR can also be calculated using the MDRD (Modification of Diet in Renal Disease) or the Cockcroft-Gault equation. As before, these methods may overestimate GFR.[19]

Radioisotope scans like EDTA or DTPA can be used to provide a more reliable GFR.[5,20] These involve injection of the radioisotope and is followed by blood samples at two, three and four hours to measure tracer elimination. When there is considerable discrepancy in size between the two kidneys on USS, the divided renal function is measured by combining the EDTA GFR with a DMSA scan.[5] The latter scan is performed three hours after the radioisotope is injected.

It has been shown that the mean GFR in young adults is 103 ml/min/1.73 m^2.[5] A reduction of about 1 ml/min/1.73 m^2 is observed in every year after the age of 40.[19] The acceptable GFR by donor age is shown in Table 4. A minimum predicted GFR of 37.5 ml/min/1.73 m^2 is advisable at the age of 80.[5]

Table 4: Acceptable GFR by donor age before donation.[5]

Donor age	Acceptable GFR
≤ 40	86
50	77
60	68
70	59
80	50

Angiography

Conventional intra-arterial angiography has largely been superseded by Magnetic Resonance Angiography (MRA) or Computer Tomography Angiography (CTA), both of which are less invasive, less expensive and can be performed faster.[5]

CTA may be less accurate in detecting small accessory arteries but MRA avoids ionizing radiation and uses smaller doses of contrast.[5,23]

Donor age

The continuing shortage of donors requires constant re-appraisal of donor criteria. In an effort to increase the donor pool, older donors have been used for living transplantation. A review of the live-donor renal transplants performed between October 2000 and September 2005 was performed at our institution. The study compared patient and renal graft survival, at one year after transplantation, between the older (age ≥ 55) and the younger (age < 55) living donors undergoing mini-open nephrectomy.

Data from 92 live-donor transplants were collected. There were 33 donors ≥ 55 years old, of which 18 were male and 15 female. 59 patients were < 55 years old, of which 32 were male and 27 were female. There was no donor perioperative morbidity or mortality in either group. Both patient and graft survival were 100% at one year in both groups. Median serum creatinine at one year was 141 μmol/l in the older group and 131 μmol/l in the younger group. There was no statistical difference between the two groups ($p = 0.053$). Median estimated creatinine clearance at one year was 57 ml/min in the older group and 62 ml/min in the younger group. There was no statistical difference between the two groups ($p = 0.131$). In view of the shortage of organs, older donors, when screened properly, seem to be a useful source of organs and a solution to the problem without increasing the operative risk or compromising graft outcome. A number of other studies have shown similar results.[24–26]

Obesity

Another way of expanding the donor pool is by performing donor nephrectomy in obese patients, that is, patients with a body mass index (BMI) of greater than 30 kg/m^2. A further study from our institution compared the time taken to remove the kidney, the total operative time, the length of the incision and the warm ischaemic time (WIT) in obese versus non-obese living donors undergoing mini-open donor nephrectomy between December 2005 and February 2007.

Some 63 patients were analysed. Sixteen patients had a BMI of greater than 30 (range = 30.5–44.8 kg/m^2, four male, 12 female). There was no statistical difference between the two groups and the time taken to remove the kidney ($p = 0.693$), the total operation time ($p = 0.788$), the length of incision ($p = 0.08$) and WIT ($p = 0.261$). This shows that fit, obese donors are a useful source of organs without necessarily increasing the operative time or the length of incision. In a study from the Mayo Clinic, Rochester, operative time was increased in patients with a BMI > 35 kg/m^2 undergoing laparoscopic donor nephrectomy, when compared with patients with a BMI < 25 kg/m^2.[27] On the whole, they had more postoperative complications but similar rate of major complications and similar hospital length-of-stay. Kidney function, up to one year of follow up, was similar in obese and non-obese donors.[27] The BTS guidelines regard a BMI > 35 kg/m^2 as an absolute contraindication and a BMI > 30 kg/m^2 as a relative contraindication and suggest a careful evaluation to identify any co-morbidity.[5] These, as well as the Amsterdam Forum guidelines also suggest advising the donor to lose weight prior to surgery and discussing the increased risk associated with donation.[5,19]

Table 5: Summaries of the different types of donor nephrectomy.

Type of nephrectomy
Open
Open donor nephrectomy
Mini-open donor nephrectomy or finger-assisted donor nephrectomy
Laparoscopic
Pure laparoscopic donor nephrectomy
Hand-assisted laparoscopic donor nephrectomy
Robotic pure laparoscopic donor nephrectomy
Robotic hand-assisted laparoscopic donor nephrectomy

Donor nephrectomy

Currently, there are a number of different ways of performing a donor nephrectomy. These can be summarized as open or laparoscopic procedures. The different types of these operations are summarized in Table 5.

Open donor nephrectomy

The traditional open kidney donation is performed through a 15–20 cm loin incision.[7] The patient is placed in the lateral decubitus position and the table is flexed. An incision is made between the eleventh and twelfth rib or just below the twelfth rib and extended anteriorly. The lower rib can be removed if necessary to improve access but this is done less often now. The Gerota's facia is then opened, followed by dissection between the perinephric fat and the kidney. The vessels are then dissected as well as the ureter with its surrounding tissue. The ureter is then clipped and divided distally. The renal artery is then clumped first, followed by the renal vein. These are then divided and the kidney removed. The vessels are either ligated with 0 vicryl suture or oversewn with prolene suture. After meticulous haemostasis, the wound is closed with number 1 loop PDS in two or three layers. 2/0 vicryl suture is applied to the fat and 3/0 vicryl or dexon subcutaneously. 40 ml of 0.25% bupivacaine is given as local anaesthetic.

Mini-open donor nephrectomy (MODN)

Mini or finger-assisted open donor nephrectomy requires similar positioning as the traditional open nephrectomy. Moreover, it involves performing a small loin incision with no rib resection. Retraction is accomplished using two 2.5 cm hand-held wound retractors and the surgeon's index and middle finger. The lead surgeon also uses a headlight with 2.5 × magnification loupes.

The Gerota's facia is then opened, followed by dissection between the perinephric fat and the kidney. Dissection continues in the same way as the open procedure but incorporates a linear articulated stapling device (ETS-Flex 35 mm, Articulating, Endoscopic Linear Cutter, Ethicon Endo-Surgery, Inc, Cincinnati, OH) for dividing the ureter, artery and vein (Figs. 1–3).

After checking for haemostasis we apply a haemostatic powder around the renal bed (ARISTA™, Medafor, Minneapolis, USA). The wound is then closed 1 loop PDS three layers. 2/0 vicryl suture is applied to the fat and 3/0 vicryl subcutaneously. 20 ml of 0.5% bupivacaine is given as local anaesthetic.

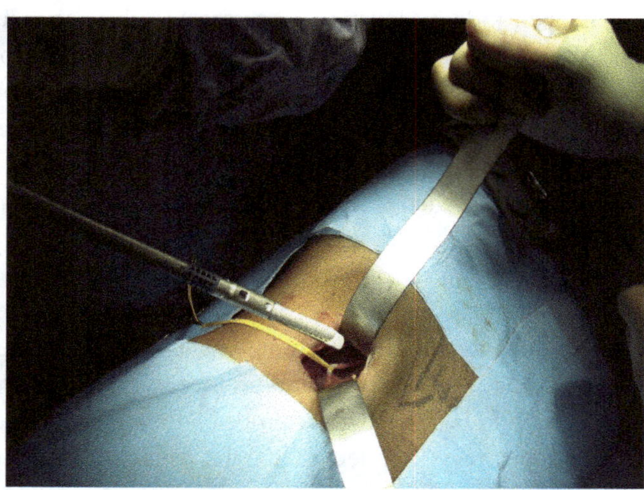

Figure 1: Ligation of left ureter with articulating, endoscopic linear cutter.

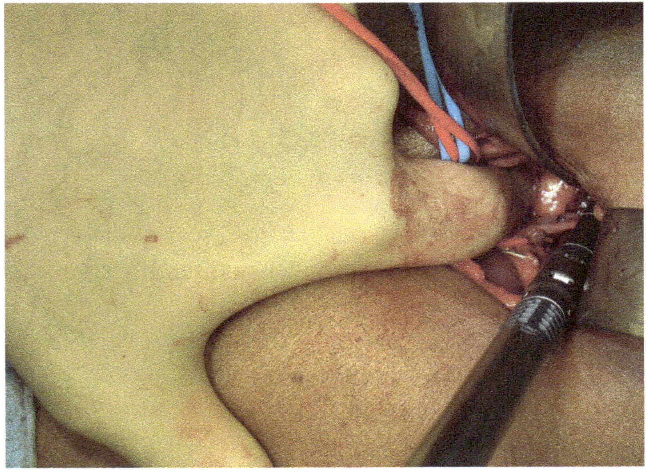

Figure 2: Ligation of left renal artery with articulating, endoscopic linear cutter.

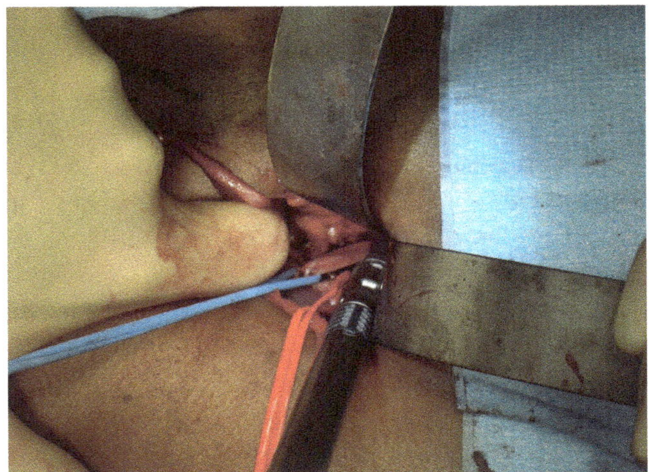

Figure 3: Ligation of left renal vein with articulating, endoscopic linear cutter.

The disadvantage of using the stabling device is the loss of 0.5 to 1 cm of vessel length. This is not usually a major problem but it becomes more significant when the right kidney has been retrieved. The main advantage of the mini-approach is that it combines a small incision (sometimes smaller than the incision from a hand-assisted or pure laparoscopic procedure) with the benefits of the laparoscopic instruments to retrieve the kidney efficiently and quickly.

Hand-assisted laparoscopic donor nephrectomy

The patient is placed in the lateral decubitus position and the table is flexed. For a left nephrectomy, an upper-midline incision is performed, the size of the surgeon's hand (7–8 cm)[28] to allow insertion of a hand port like Gelport™ (Applied Medical, CA, USA). For a right nephrectomy a lower-midline or a pfannenstiel incision is carried out. Two further 12 mm incisions are made on the lateral aspect of the abdomen to allow insertion of the laparoscope, which is attached to a video camera, and the hand piece of the harmonic scalpel® system (Ethicon Endo-Surgery, Inc, Cincinnati, OH). Dissection can be transperitonealy or retroperitonealy.[20,29] In the former procedure the dissection commences by reflecting the left colon medially along the white line. In the latter procedure the peritoneum is separated from the rest of the abdominal wall using hand dissection. This avoids the mobilization of the colon, spleen or splenocolic ligament. Dissection around the vessels and the kidney continues. The left gonadal vein, as well as the adrenal vein on the same side, is always divided in this procedure whereas this may not be necessary in the mini-open donor nephrectomy where dissection may be closer to the hilum. LigaSure™ (Valleylab, a division of Tyco Healthcare Group LP, Colorado, USA) can be used to divide these vessels. The ureter is then clipped and divided distally at the pelvic brim. A linear articulated stapling device (ETS-Flex 35 mm, Articulating, Endoscopic Linear Cutter, Ethicon Endo-Surgery, Inc, Cincinnati, OH) is used for dividing the renal artery and vein. The kidney is then extracted through the Gelport™. The main wound is closed with 1 loop PDS and an absorbable subcutaneous suture. The deep part of the port wounds is closed with 2/0 vicryl and the superficial part with 3/0 vicryl or dexon. 20 ml of 0.5% bupivacaine is given as local anaesthetic.

There have been a number of publications over the last few years showing that hand-assisted laparoscopic donor nephrectomy has a number of advantages when compared to the traditional open donor nephrectomy including minimal morbidity,[28–32] reduction in hospital stay and analgesia requirements as well as earlier return to work.[28] Long-term graft function is similar after both procedures. Disadvantages include increase in operative time.[28] The length of the warm ischemic time is more in some studies[28] but less in others.[29]

When compared with the pure laparoscopic nephrectomy, the hand-assisted procedure has the advantage of extra safety and security for controlling bleeding[33–35] as well as reduction in operating time, quick kidney retrieval and reduction in warm ischemic time.[29]

Pure laparoscopic donor nephrectomy

Pure laparoscopic donor nephrectomy was first described by Ratner *et al.* in 1995 at Johns Hopkins University School of Medicine, Baltimore, Maryland, USA.[36] This procedure is considered more demanding than the equivalent hand-assisted operation.[28] It involves similar positioning of the patient as described above. Dissection can be transperitoneally or retroperitoneally,[37] as in the hand-assisted laparoscopic operation, but the former way is the most commonly carried out procedure.[38,39]

Four ports are established.[40,41] The laparoscope is primarily introduced through the umbilical port and the main dissecting instruments through the epigastric and iliac fossa ports. The colon is mobilized prior to opening the Gerota's facia medially. The upper pole is usually dissected first[38,40] to allow the kidney to dissent. Dissecting the posteriolateral attachments at a later stage prevents twisting of the kidney around the vessels.[40] The renal vein and artery are then freed as well as the ureter. The tissue between the ureter and lower pole is preserved to reduce the risk of disrupting its blood supply. A 6 cm pfannensteil incision[39] is then made down to the peritoneum. A small cut is made through this to allow an edoscopic bag (Endocatch, US Surgical, Norwalk, CT, USA)[37] into the abdominal cavity. The kidney is positioned into the bag prior to dividing the vessels with an endovascular stapler. Once this is done the bag is closed and removed. The kidney is then flushed with preservation fluid and cooled down as normal. The pneumopritoneum is re-established to check for haemostasis.[40] The wound is closed with 1 loop PDS and an absorbable subcutaneous suture. The deep part of the port wounds is closed with 2/0 vicryl and superficial part with 3/0 vicryl or dexon. Local anaesthetic is used as above.

Hand-assisted and pure laparoscopic donor nephrectomy are safe procedures as shown by groups that have done more than 1,000 such operations.[42] Other advantages over the traditional open procedure include less postoperative pain, less in-hospital stay and earlier return to work when compared with the open procedure.[28,35,37–40,43] A number of randomized trials have also confirmed the above advantages.[44–47]

A meta-analysis comparing hand-assisted versus laparoscopic live-donor nephrectomy showed both operations to have similar complication rates but the hand-assisted procedure was associated with shorter operative and warm ischemic time and less intraoperative bleeding.[48]

Rombotic live-donor nephrectomy

Robotic (Da Vinci Surgical System, Intuitive Surgical, Mountain View, CA) hand-assisted or laparoscopic donor nephrectomy are procedures performed more commonly in the USA.[49,50] The main difference of the robotic approach is that the surgeon sits at the console and the assistant by the side of the patient, scrubbed.[41] In the hand-assisting operation the assistant has his hand inside the Gelport™ and in the laparoscopic procedure he or she uses instruments through the umbilical port. It is argued that it may be better than the laparoscopic procedure because of the greater freedom of movement and the use of three-dimensional vision.[49] The largest study is from the University of Illinois at the Chicago Medical Centre, Illinois, USA, where 209 procedures were performed between 2000 and 2005.[50] The technique is reported to be safe and effective[50] even though there is a long learning curve.

Donor risks

Complications related to all types of nephrectomies are described in Table 6. These are divided into short-term and long-term risks.

Early complications after laparoscopic nephrectomy vary from 0% to 30%.[51] These rates are similar to the ones observed after open donor nephrectomy (0–35%).[51] Chronic wound pain is more frequent after

Table 6: Descriptions of the risks to the donor.

Short-term risks	Long-term risks
Morbidity	Morbidity
• Bleeding	• Incisional hernia
• Re-operation	• Wound pain (chronic)
• Urinary track infection	• Small bowel obstruction
• Chest infection	• Hypertension
• Wound infection	• Proteinuria
• Haematoma	• Deterioration of renal function
• Seroma	
• Testicular pain	
• Wound pain (postoperative)	
• Wound dehiscence	
• Ureteric complications	
• Ileus	
• Deep vein thrombosis	
• Pulmonary embolus	
• Pneumothorax	
• Injury to neighbouring structures (e.g. spleen, bowel)	
• Conversion to open procedure (Laparoscopic procedures only)	
• Urinary retention	
Mortality	

open nephrectomy.[51–53] Pneumothorax used to be more common after open nephterctomy[53,54] but has now been reduced with the adoption of the newer procedures. At the end of MODN we always check for a pneumothorax. This is done by adding normal saline in the renal bed cavity, expanding the lungs fully for a few seconds and observing for bubbles. If a pneumothorax is observed, a small feeding tube is inserted into the pleural cavity and suction is applied. This is than slowly removed as the hole is closed with a 2/0 vicryl purse string. A postoperative chest X-ray is performed.

Testicular pain seems to be more frequent after laparoscopic live-donor surgery at about 3%.[55] Ureteric complications used to be more common in the first few years of starting laparoscopic surgery. Dissection medial to the gonadal vein and preservation of the fatty tissue in the triangle between the proximal and distal ureter and the lower pole of the kidney has now reduced the number of complications.[28,41]

Conversion from a laparoscopic operation to an open procedure varies from 0.2% to 2.8%.[56] This improves with experience. The risk for a major complication[5,17] is 2% and the risk of death is 0.03%.[5,17,18] Severe bleeding is a rare complication after nephrectomy but can be fatal.[54] Surgical clips are associated with the most risk whereas suture or staple transfixion is the safest way of securing the renal vessels.[54]

Delmonico *et al.* presented the outcome of 10,828 living-donor nephrectomies performed between 1999 and 2001 in the USA.[57] Some 52.3% were open, 20.7% hand-assisted and 27% pure laparoscopic procedures. Two donors (0.02%) died, one after hand-assisted laparoscopic nephrectomy from pulmonary embolus and one after laparoscopic nephrectomy for unspecified reasons. A third patient was in a persistent vegetative state after hypotension secondary to intraoperative bleeding during pure laparoscopic operation.[57] Despite these results it is well known that live kidney donors go on to live longer than the general population of the same age.[17] This is probably due to the rigorous selection process that selects the fittest donors.

Longer-term risks include hypertension, proteinuria and reduction renal function. With respect to hypertension, the donor has a risk of raised blood pressure by 10 mmHg at ten years after the operation.[58] With respect to proteinuria, a meta-analysis of 42 studies showed a pooled incidence of protein in the urine of 12%.[59] The same paper showed the pooled donor GFR to be 10 ml/min/1.73 m^2 lower after surgery compared with controls.[59] Because of the risk of these complications patient are followed up yearly after nephrectomy. Moreover, after transperitoneal laparoscopic surgery there is a small risk of bowel obstruction secondary to adhesions.[57]

Donor outcome

Critical factors in donor nephrectomy are absolute donor safety and provision of a high-quality allograft. Minimizing donor morbidity is also

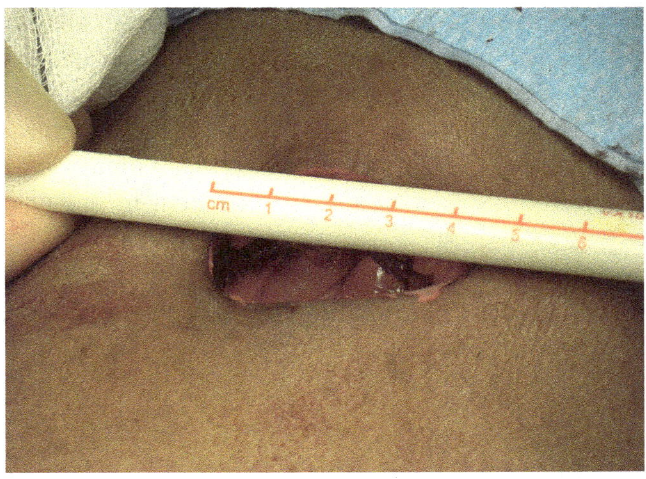

Figure 4: Measurement of incision length just before wound closure.

important, particularly decreasing wound pain and achieving a small cosmetic scar. Mini-open (MODN) and laparoscopic donor nephrectomy aim to achieve these goals. We prospectively audited our MODN series.[59] In the year between 2005 and 2006 two surgeons performed 71 MODN (46 female, 25 male). The left kidney was harvested in 61 cases. The mean patient body mass index (BMI) was 27 (range 17.5 to 44). The mean skin incision length was 6.6 cm (range 4.5–9.5 cm, Fig. 4), the kidney out time 77.5 minutes (range 30–150 mins), the operative time 119 minutes (range 50–210 mins), the warm ischemia time 4 minutes (range 1.5–10 mins), estimated blood loss 110 mls (range 20–450 mls) and length of postoperative hospital stay 5.2 days (range 3–8 days). Some eight donors had multiple renal arteries on the donor kidney as predicted on preoperative MRA. Two arterial vascular anastomoses were required in 15 recipients and three in one recipient.[59]

Some six donors had minor postoperative complications. These were one respiratory infection, one fast atrial fibrillation, one ileus (despite a retroperitoneal approach), one urinary infection and one urinary retention. All recipients had primary graft function except one recipient who required graft nephrectomy on day four after operation for renal vein thrombosis.[59] There was no mortality.

The above findings show that MODN can be performed safely via a small retroperitoneal incision of similar size as the one used to retrieve a donor kidney laparoscopically. This technique is applicable to almost all potential donors regardless of BMI. MODN provides excellent grafts for transplantation and has allowed us to expand our living-donor program such that now over 70% of renal transplantation in our unit is living donation.

Similar to the mini-open donor nephrectomy, all varieties of laparoscopic donor nephrectomy are also safe procedures that result in a small number of complications, reduced postoperative pain, short in-hospital stay and early return to work.[28,35,37–40,43–47]

Ways of expanding the living-donor pool

Over the last few years a number of different methods have been adopted in an attempt to expand the donor pool. In the UK, the Human Tissue Act became law in September 2006. With respect to living donation, it allows more flexibility as to who can donate to whom, so that it is not just genetic relatives and people with close personal relationships that can donate.[60] In addition, paired donation and altruistic donations are now allowed.[60] The former way allows two donors who are ABO or HLA incompatible with their two intended recipients to exchange kidneys so that they become compatible.[8,61] This allows a recipient to acquire a more compatible organ without the need, for example, for desensitization. It also prevents the donor from being lost from the live-donor pool if he or she were not allowed to donate.[61] Larger groups of donors and recipients can be created as well. The latter way of expanding the living-donor pool, allows a fit, competent person who is willing, to donate one of his or her kidneys to the living-donor pool, free of coercion and without any financial benefit.[8]

Another way of expanding the donor pool is by establishing ABO incompatible kidney transplantation programmes as well as desensitization programs.[62–64] These involve immunoadsorption, plasmapheresis, intravenous immunoglobulin administration, rituximab (anti-CD20 antibody) and powerful immunosuppression. Graft and patient outcome after these procedures are very good.[62]

Table 7: Benefits of live kidney transplantation.[16]

Benefits
Allows a planned (elective) operation to be carried out by a consultant anaesthetist and consultant surgeon.
Recipient and donor psychosocially more prepared.
Kidney anatomy already known from CT/MRA. Less likely to have injury during retrieval.
Healthy kidney chosen for retrieval.
Less stress to kidney during retrieval because of avoidance of abnormal physiology of brainstem death.
Shorter cold ischemic time.
Less delayed graft function.
Better match.
Less rejection.
Long waiting time on dialysis avoided.
Pre-emptive transplantation possible.
Better kidney and patient survival.
Less cost.
Allows more patients to be transplanted by increasing the donor pool.

Finally, by expanding the criteria for living donors, for example, allowing patients with hypertension as well as obese and elderly patients to donate, the live-donor pool can increase further.[8]

The Recipient

Recipient benefits

The two main benefits of transplantation are avoiding dialysis and therefore enhancement of quality of life, and improvement of patient survival. These as well as other important benefits to the recipient of a live-donor kidney are summarised in Table 7.

Conclusions

The transplant team needs to provide the donor with the maximum safety possible. By providing a detailed and complete evaluation of the donor, the risk of the operation will be reduced to the minimum. Guidelines and protocols should be followed in order to provide this safety to the donor.

Between 2000 and 2006, more than 2,500 live-donor operations have been performed in the UK.[65] About 25% were laparoscopic operations and the rest were open procedures.[65] There was only one death within the first year after surgery at three months after discharge. This was in the open nephrectomy group. There were five more deaths more than a year after surgery. Length of stay was significantly shorter in the laparoscopic group (4.5 vs 6). Minor morbidity was significantly less in the laparoscopic group (7.4% vs 13.3%) but major morbidity rate was similar (3.5% in both groups).[65] As laparoscopic donor nephrectomy is safe, we will certainly observe a further increase in the number of such procedures in the future; especially after the endorsement of the procedure by the National Institute for Health and Clinical Excellence in 2004.[66]

MODN is also a safe procedure with similar results such as reduced postoperative pain and cosmesis but also with other advantages such as reduced operating time. This directly benefits the patient and reduces the cost of the procedure. Donors should be followed up yearly to monitor for long-term complications such as hypertension, proteinuria and kidney dysfunction so that they can be dealt with at an early stage if it becomes necessary.

References

1. Merrill JP, Murray JE, Harrison JH, Guild WR. Successful homotransplantation of the human kidney between identical twins. *JAMA* 1956;160:277–82.
2. Merrill JP, Murray JE, Harrison JH, Guild WR. Renal homotransplantation in identical twins. *Surg. Forum* 1956;6:432–6.
3. Merrill JP, Murray JE, Harrison JH, Guild WR. Milestones in nephrology. Renal homotransplantation in identical twins. *J. Am. Soc. Nephrol.* 2001;12:201–4.
4. Woodruff MF, Robson JS, Ross JA, Nolan B, Lambie AT. Transplantation of a kidney from an identical twin. *Lancet* 1961 June 10;1:1245–9.
5. http://www.bts.org.uk/Forms/Guidelines_complete_Oct05.pdf. Accessed 23 June 2007.
6. http://www.optn.org/ar2005/. Accessed 23 June 2007.
7. Magee CC, Pascual M. Update in renal transplantation. *Arch. Intern. Med.* 2004;164:1373–88.

8. Baid-Agrawal S, Frei UA. Living-donor renal transplantation: recent developments and perspectives. *Nat. Clin. Pract.* 2007;3:31–41.
9. http://www.uktransplant.org.uk/ukt/statistics/transplant_activity_report/archive_activity_reports/pdf/ukt/2001revsd.pdf. Accessed 23 June 2007.
10. http://www.uktransplant.org.uk/ukt/statistics/transplant_activity_report/archive_activity_reports/pdf/ukt/uk_txa_2002-2003_complete.pdf. Accessed 23 June 2007.
11. http://www.uktransplant.org.uk/ukt/statistics/transplant_activity_report/archive_activity_reports/pdf/ukt/tx_activity_report_2004_uk2_complete.pdf. Accessed 23 June 2007.
12. http://www.uktransplant.org.uk/ukt/statistics/transplant_activity_report/archive_activity_reports/pdf/ukt/tx_activity_report_2005_uk_%20complete.pdf. Accessed 23 June 2007.
13. http://www.uktransplant.org.uk/ukt/statistics/transplant_activity_report/current_activity_reports/ukt/transplant_activity_uk_2005-2006.pdf. Accessed 23 June 2007.
14. Hariharan S, Johnson CP, Bresnahan BA, Taranto SE, McIntosh MJ, Stablein D. Improved graft survival after renal transplantation in the United States, 1988 to 1996. *N. Engl. J. Med.* 2000;342:605–12.
15. Terasaki PI, Cecka M, Gjertson DW, Takemoto S. High survival rates of kidney transplants from spousal and living unrelated donors. *N. Engl. J. Med.* 1995;333:333–6.
16. Weitz J, Koch M, Mehrabi A, Schemmer P, Zeier M, Beimler J, Büchler M, Schmidt J. Living-donor kidney transplantation: risks of the donor – benefits of the recipient. *Clin. Transplant.* 2006;20(17):13–16.
17. Hartmann A, Fauchald P, Westlie L, Brekke IB, Holdass H. The risk of the living kidney donation. *Nephrol. Dial. Transplant.* 2003;18:871–3.
18. Najarian JS, Chavers BM, McHugh LE, Matas AJ. Twenty years or more of follow-up of living kidney donors. *Lancet* 1992;340:807–10.
19. The Ethics Committee of the Transplantation Society. A report of the Amsterdam Forum on the care of the live kidney donor: data and medical guidelines. *Transplantation* 2005;79:S53–S66.
20. Gaston RS, Wadström J. *Living Donor Kidney Transplantation, Current Practices, Emerging Trends and Evolving Challenges*. London: Taylor & Francis. 2005.
21. Longmore M, Wilkinson I, Török E. *Oxford Handbook of Clinical Medicine* 5th edn. Oxford: Oxford University Press. 2001.

22. Provan D, Krentz A. *Oxford Handbook of Clinical and Laboratory Investigation*. Oxford: Oxford University Press. 2002.
23. Rankin SC, Jan W, Koffman CG. Non-invasive imaging of living related kidney donors: evaluation with CT angiography and gadolinium-enhanced MR angiography. *AJR Am. J. Roentgenol.* 2001;177:349–55.
24. Wolters HH, Schmidt-Traub H, Holzen HJ, Suwelack B, Dietl KH, Senninger N, Brockmann JG. Living-donor kidney transplantation from the elderly donor. *Transplant. Proc.* 2006;38:659–60.
25. Johnson SR, Khwaja K, Pavlakis M, Monaco AP, Hanto DW. Older living donors provide excellent quality kidneys: a single centre experience (older living donors). *Clin. Transplant.* 2005;5:600–6.
26. Sahin S, Manga Sahin G, Turkmen A, Sever MS. Utilization of elderly donors in living related kidney transplantation. *Transplant. Proc.* 2006;38:385–7.
27. Heimbach JK, Taler SJ, Prieto M, Cosio FG, Textor SC, Kudva YC, Chow GK, Ishitani MB, Larson TS, Stegall MD. Obesity in living kidney donors: clinical characteristics and outcomes in the era of laparoscopic donor nephrectomy. *Am. J. Transplant.* 2005;5:1057–64.
28. Challacombe B, Mamode N. Laparoscopic live-donor nephrectomy. *Nephrol. Dial. Transplant.* 2004;19:2961–4.
29. Wadström J, Lindström P. Hand-assisted retroperitoneoscopic living-donor nephrectomy: initial ten cases. *Transplantation* 2002;73:1839–41.
30. Kercher K, Dahl D, Harland R, Blute R, Gallagher K, Litwin D. Hand-assisted laparoscopic donor nephrectomy minimizes warm ischemia. *Urology* 2001;58:152–6.
31. Chiong E, Yip SK, Cheng WS, Vathsala A, Li MK. Hand-assisted laparoscopic living-donor nephrectomy. *Ann. Acad. Med. Singapore* 2004;33:294–7.
32. Salazar A, Pelletier R, Yilmaz S, Monroy-Cuadros M, Tibbles LA, McLaughlin K, Sepandj F. Use of a minimally invasive donor nephrectomy programme to select technique for live-donor nephrectomy. *Am. J. Surg.* 2005;189:558–62.
33. Lai IR, Tsai MK, Lee PH. Hand-assisted versus total laparoscopic live-donor nephrectomy. *J. Formos Med. Assoc.* 2004;103:749–53.
34. Velidedeoglu E, Williams N, Brayman KL, Desai NM, Campos L, Palanjian M, Wocjik M, Bloom R, Grossman RA, Mange K, Barker CF, Naji A, Markmann JF. Comparison of open, laparoscopic, and hand-assisted approaches to live-donor nephrectomy. *Transplantation* 2002;74:169–72.

35. Stekas G, Papalois VE, Mitsis M, Hakim NS. Laparoscopic live-donor nephrectomy: a step forward in kidney transplantation? *JSLS* 2003;7:197–206.
36. Ratner LE, Ciseck LJ, Moore RG, Cigarroa FG, Kaufman HS, Kavoussi LR. *Transplantation* 1995;60:1047–9.
37. Lind MY, Ijzermans JNM, Bonjer HJ. Open vs laparoscopic donor nephrectomy. Open vs laparoscopic donor nephrectomy in renal transplantation. *BJU Int.* 2002;89:162–8.
38. Noguira M, Kavoussi LR, Bhayani SB. Laparoscopic live-donor nephrectomy: current status. *BJU Int.* 2005;95(2):59–64.
39. Giessing M. Laparoscopic living-donor nephrectomy. *Nephrol. Dial. Transplant.* 2004;19(4):iv36–iv40.
40. Waller JR, Hiley AL, Mullin EJ, Veitch PS, Nicholson ML. Living kidney donation: a comparison of laparoscopic and conventional open operations. *Postgrad. Med. J.* 2002;78:153–7.
41. Humar A, Matas A, Payne WD. *Atlas of Organ Transplantation*. London: Springer. 2006.
42. Cooper M, Al-Qudah HS, Jacobs SC, Phelan M, Nogueira JM, Philosophe B, Bartlett ST. Laparoscopic donor nephrectomy for transplantation: ten years and 1,000 consecutive cases. *Am. J. Transplant.* 2006; 6(2):286.
43. Lennerling A, Blohmé I, Östraat Ö, Lönroth H, Olausson M, Nyberg G. Laparoscopic or open surgery for living-donor nephrectomy. *Nephrol. Dial. Transplant.* 2001;16:383–6.
44. Oyen O, Anderson M, Mathisen L, *et al.* Laparoscopic versus open living-donor nephrectomy: experiences from a prospective, randomized, single-centre study focusing on donor safety. *Transplantation* 2005;79:1236–40.
45. Wolf JS, Merion RM, Leichtman AB, *et al.* Randomized controlled trial of hand-assisted laparoscopic versus open surgical live-donor nephrectomy. *Transplantation* 2001;72:284–90.
46. Simforoosh N, Basiri A, Tabibi A, *et al.* Comparison of laparoscopic and open donor nephrectomy: a randomized controlled trial. *BJU Int.* 2005;95:851–5.
47. Lewis GR, Brook NR, Waller JR, *et al.* A comparison of traditional open, minimal-incision donor nephrectomy and laparoscopic donor nephrectomy. *Transpl. Int.* 2004;17:589–95.
48. Kokkinos C, Nanidis T, Antcliffe D, Darzi AW, Tekkis P, Papalois V. Comparison of laparoscopic versus hand-assisted live-donor nephrectomy. *Transplantation* 2007;83:41–7.

49. Horgan S, Vanuno D, Sileri P, Cicalese L, Benedetti E. Robotic-assisted laparoscopic donor nephrectomy for kidney transplantation. *Transplantation* 2002;73:1474–9.
50. Gorodner V, Horgan S, Galvani C, Manzelli A, Oberholzer J, Sankary H, Testa G, Benedetti E. Routine left robotic-assisted laparoscopic donor nephrectomy is safe and effective regardless of the presence of vascular anomalies. *Transpl. Int.* 2006;19:636–40.
51. Handschin AE, Weber M, Demartines N, Clavien P-A. Laparoscopic donor nephrectomy. *BJS* 2003;90:1323–32.
52. Buell JF, Lee L, Martin JE, Dake NA, Cavanaugh TM, Hanaway MJ, Weiskittel P, Munda R, Alexander JW, Cardi M, Peddi VR, Zavala EY, Berilla E, Clippard M, First MR, Woodle ES. Laparoscopic donor nephrectomy vs open live-donor nephrectomy: a quality of life and functional study. *Clin. Transplant.* 2005;19:102–9.
53. Shaffer D, Sahyoun AI, Madras PN, Monaco AP. Two hundred and one consecutive living-donor nephrectomies. *Arch. Surg.* 1998;133:426–31.
54. Friedman AL, Peters TG, Jones KW, Boulware LE, Ratner LE. Fatal and non-fatal hemorrhagic complications of living kidney donation. *Ann. Surg.* 2006;243:126–30.
55. Brook NR, Harper SJ, Waller JR, Nicholson ML. A consecutive series of 70 laparoscopic donor nephrectomies demonstrates the safety of this new operation. *Transplant. Proc.* 2005;37:627–8.
56. Melcher ML, Carter JT, Posselt A, Duh QY, Stoller M, Freise CE, Kang SM. More than 500 consecutive laparoscopic donor nephrectomies without conversion or repeated surgery. *Arch. Surg.* 2005;140:835–9.
57. Matas AJ, Bartlett ST, Leichtman AB, Delmonico FL. Morbidity and mortality after living kidney donation, 1999–2001:survey of United States transplant centres. *Am. J. Transplant.* 2003;3:830–4.
58. Boudville N, Prasad GV, Knoll G, Muirhead N, Thiessen-Philbrook H, Yang RC, Rosas-Arellano MP, Housawi A, Garg AX. Donor Nephrectomy Outcomes Research (DONOR) Network. Meta-analysis: risk for hypertension in living kidney donors. *Ann. Intern. Med.* 2006;145:185–96.
59. Dosani T, Olsburgh J, Mustafa N, Kessaris N, Papalois V, Hakim N. Key-hole mini-open donor nephrectomy: a single institution experience. *Am. J. Transplant.* 2007;7(2):489.

60. www.hta.gov.uk/about_hta/human_tissue_act.cfm. Accessed 29 August 2006.
61. Mahendran AO, Veitch PS. Paired-exchange programmes can expand the live kidney donor pool. *BJS* 2007;94:657–64.
62. Tyden G, Donauer J, Wadstrom J, Kumlien G, Wilpert J, Nilsson T, Genberg H, Pisarski P, Tufveson G. Implementation of a protocol for ABO-incompatible kidney transplantation – a three-centre experience with 60 consecutive transplantations. *Transplantation* 2007;83:1153–5.
63. Schwartz J, Stegall MD, Kremers WK, Gloor J. Complications, resource utilization, and cost of ABO-incompatible living-donor kidney transplantation. *Transplantation* 2006;82:155–63.
64. Beimler JH, Susal C, Zeier M. Desensitization strategies enabling successful renal transplantation in highly sensitized patients. *Clin. Transplant.* 2006; 20(17):7–12.
65. Mamode N, Hadjianastassiou V, Cacciola R, Johnson R. How safe is laparoscopic donor nephrectomy in the United Kingdom? Data from the UK Transplant Registry in 2,509 patients. Oral presentation (O10), BTS, Manchester, 2007.
66. http://guidance.nice.org.uk/IPG57. Accessed 12 August 2007.

Chapter 3

Live-Donor Liver Transplantation in Adults

Sheung Tat Fan and Chi Leung Liu

History

Liver transplantation is the most successful treatment method for patients with end-stage liver disease. The rapid increase in the number of potential recipients on the waiting list in the 80s largely exceeded the number of brain-dead organ donors available. Apart from increasing the use of marginal quality brain-dead donor grafts, transplant surgeons explored the feasibility of donation of partial liver grafts from living persons. On 8 December 1988, Raia *et al.*[1] made the first attempt at live-donor liver transplantation (LDLT) in a four and a half-year-old girl suffering from biliary atresia. They made the second attempt on 21 July 1989. Although the two donors recovered uneventfully from segments II and III (Couinaud classification[2]) donation surgery, both recipients could not survive the transplant operations. In July 1989, Strong *et al.*[3] performed the first successful LDLT in an 11-month-old boy using a segments II and III graft donated by his mother. The operation was rapidly adopted by many liver transplant centres around the world. This surgical innovation has significantly reduced the mortality rate of children waiting for liver transplantation and provided the only source of organs for transplantation in countries where cadaveric organ donation is prohibited. The demand for liver transplantation was, however, much higher in adults than in children. In 1991, Haberal *et al.*[4] extended LDLT to adult recipients (age > 18). Thus, in his early series, he transplanted left-liver grafts to eight patients, seven of whom suffered from chronic liver diseases. On 2 November 1993, Makuuchi *et al.*[5] performed the first successful adult-to-adult LDLT in the world using a left-liver graft. The recipient was a 53-year-old female patient suffering from primary biliary cirrhosis and the donor was her 25-year-old son. The left-liver graft, including the middle hepatic vein (MHV), weighed 404 gm, which was 42% of the estimated ideal liver mass for the recipient. Both the donor and recipient recovered from the operations. On 12 July 1994, we performed a similar operation in a married couple.[6] The recipient, aged 26 and weighing 59 kg, suffered from fulminant hepatic failure of unknown etiology. The donor was her husband, who weighed 82 kg. The graft weighed 623 gm, which was about 43% of the estimated standard liver mass for the recipient.[7] The recipient recovered without any neurological deficit and the donor has remained well ever since the operation.

Left-liver LDLT, however, is quite limited in clinical application because the left-liver graft volume is generally small and a much heavier donor is required to donate a sufficiently large left-liver graft to a small adult recipient. Such donor-recipient match is uncommon, especially in Asia, where most of the hepatitis B sufferers are male. Makuuchi *et al.*[8] advocated inclusion of the caudate lobe in the left-liver graft. Such inclusion may increase the graft volume by 3–8%.[9] However, the limitation is the capacity of the upper abdomen of the small recipient in accommodating a large left-liver graft. After portal vein reperfusion and expansion of the left-liver graft, exposure of the liver hilum for hepatic artery and bilio-enteric reconstruction is difficult, especially when the space between the costal arch and spine is limited. To expose the liver hilum, the liver graft will be compressed against the costal arch rendering the caudal part of the liver graft ischemic.[10] Therefore, the volume of the functioning liver mass would be less than expected. A right-liver graft, on the other hand, situated in the spacious right subphrenic cavity is devoid of injury during implantation and on wound closure. In May 1996, we performed the first successful right-liver LDLT in an adult[11] (Fig. 1). Right-liver LDLT was rapidly adopted in many liver transplant centres around the world. It increases the salvage rate of patients waiting for deceased donor liver grafts, especially in emergency situations.

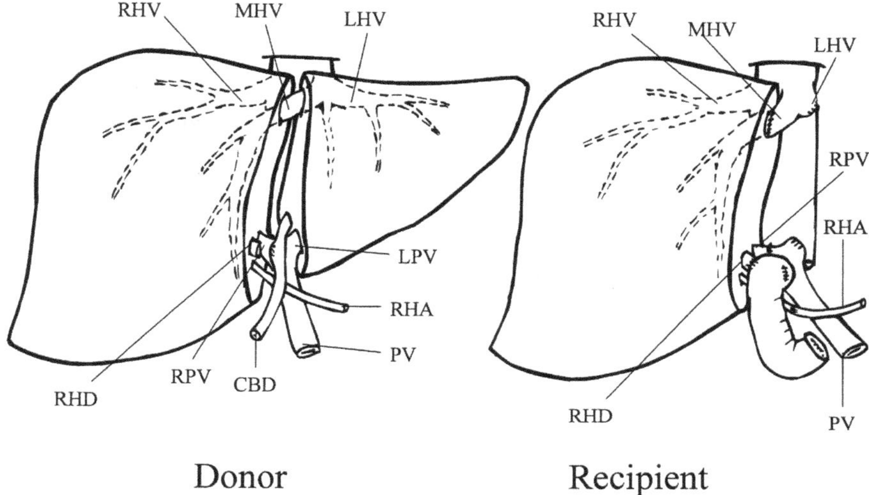

Figure 1: Diagram showing adult-to-adult live-donor liver transplantation including the middle hepatic vein.

In this chapter, we will present our experience and current technique of LDLT in adults and discuss the pertinent controversies.

Donor Evaluation

Only completely healthy persons aged between 18 and 55 are accepted for organ donation. History of diabetes mellitus, hypertension, ischemic heart disease, malignancy and mental disorders preclude the candidacy of donation. Obese people (BMI > 30 kg/m^2) are more likely to have cardiovascular and respiratory co-morbidities and fatty liver. Thorough investigation including a liver biopsy must be carried out before they are considered for donation. Any person with a history of peptic ulcer disease mandates upper endoscopy. Female potential donors of reproductive age and who are sexually active should undergo a pregnancy test. The use of oral contraceptive pills or hormonal devices indicates perioperative deep vein thrombosis prophylaxis by subcutaneous heparin in addition to physical means. It is arguable whether a person with a history of tuberculosis completing a full course of drug treatment is suitable for donation.

The issue is relevant to Asia where tuberculosis is common. The data on this issue are few but there is a possibility of transmitting an occult source of tuberculosis to the recipient.[12] Moreover, reactivation of tuberculosis after a major hepatectomy in the donor is not impossible and constitutes a real risk when the regenerated liver could not handle the anti-tuberculosis drugs. To evaluate the potential donor thoroughly, it is advisable to construct a checklist and questionnaire of all the aforementioned items.

Once the recipient is accepted on the waiting list, it is our practice to provide a pamphlet containing information about liver transplantation to the patient and their family. The patient is free to choose between the options of LDLT and deceased-donor liver transplantation (DDLT). Once a volunteer opts for live donation, the process of pre-transplant evaluation will begin.

The potential donor will go through critical evaluations that consist of medical history and physical examination, haematology, biochemistry and serology tests. The latter consists of hepatitis B and C, HIV and cytomegalovirus serology. An unexpected coagulation disorder resulting in severe pulmonary embolism has occurred in a donor.[13] Systemic screening for coagulation disorder is then suggested for thorough evaluation of donors.[13] Such practice is expensive and the cost-effectiveness has not been established. Nevertheless, any donor with a history of coagulation disorder should call for thorough screening for prothrombotic states.

If all the assessments show that the potential donor is suitable, he/she will be assessed by a clinical psychologist. The clinical psychologist plays an important role in assessing the suitability of donation. He/she will interview the donor and recipient independently and collect the following information:

1. Clinical observation of the potential donor.
2. Relevant background.
3. Events leading to the proposed organ transplant.
4. The psychological condition of the intended donor.
5. The intended donor's reason for his/her decision to donate the organ.
6. The relationship and/or emotional ties between the intended donor and intended recipient.

Based on the information, the clinical psychologist makes an independent recommendation as to whether the donor is suitable to undergo donation. In his/her report, for the purpose of medicolegal requirement and documentation, it is preferred that he/she makes the following statements:

1. The intended donor's decision to donate the organ is made voluntarily.
2. The intended donor is psychologically prepared for both the removal and transplant operations.
3. The intended donor has adequate ability to understand what is involved in donating the organ.
4. There are no specific difficulties in communicating with the intended donor.
5. The intended donor has understood that he/she has given his/her consent to removal of the organ without coercion or offer of inducement.
6. The intended donor understood his/her entitlement to withdraw consent at any time.
7. The intended donor has received the relevant information pamphlet about organ donation and transplantation.
8. The doctor-in-charge of the intended donor has explained to him/her the nature, implications, possible postoperative complications and long-term effects of the procedures.
9. The doctor-in-charge of the intended donor has explained to him/her the mortality rate for the organ donation surgery would be 0.5%.
10. The doctor-in-charge of the intended donor has explained to him/her the mortality rate for the transplant surgery for the recipient would be 15%.

Following the clinical psychologist's assessment that the donor is suitable for donation, computed tomography (CT) under sodium bicarbonate cover[14] is performed. The main objective of the CT is to detect parenchymal disease, to study the vascular anatomy and to perform liver volumetry. By three-dimensional reconstruction, it is possible to obtain a clear picture of vascular anatomy at the liver hilum. For right-liver LDLT, it is important to identify the origin of the segment IV hepatic artery, which must be protected during donor operation. For left-liver LDLT, the origin and the number of branches of the left hepatic artery are examined. The presence of two left hepatic arteries is not a contraindication for left-liver LDLT because, technically, it is possible to reconstruct two hepatic arteries under microscope. Not infrequently, the two hepatic arteries communicate with each other, rendering only one hepatic artery reconstruction necessary.[15] The hepatic vein anatomy could also be studied thoroughly by three-dimensional reconstruction on the CT scan. For right-liver donation, the focus of examination is the MHV and its receiving branches, especially at the junction with the left hepatic vein or inferior vena cava (IVC). If the MHV is to be included in the right-liver graft, the segment IVb hepatic vein joining the root of MHV should be preserved in order to maximize venous drainage of segment IV and liver function of the donor[16] (Fig. 2). Sometimes, a large trunk joining the MHV is the combined segments IV and III hepatic vein. Sacrifice of such branch will definitely lead to donor liver failure. Segment IVb hepatic vein draining into the left

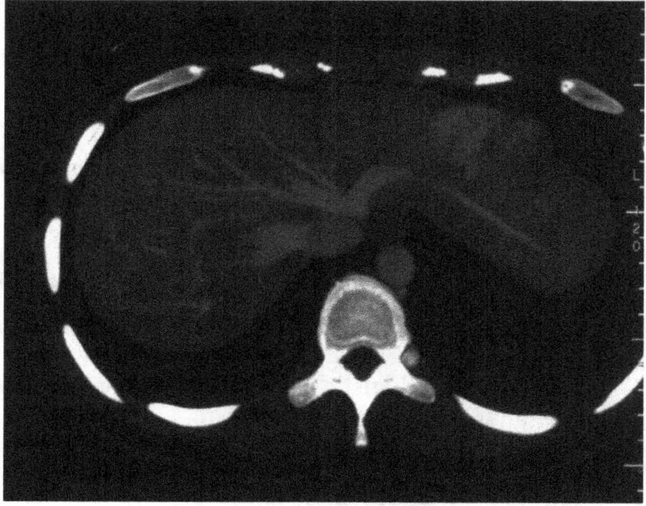

Figure 2: Computed tomography scan showing a segment IVb hepatic vein (arrow) which could be protected during donor operation by dividing the middle hepatic vein proximal to it (dotted line).

hepatic vein is the most favorable condition for right-liver donation including the MHV.[17] Major segment VIII hepatic vein near to the root of the MHV is obvious on a CT scan and must be preserved whether the MHV is to be included in the right-liver graft or not. In the case of left-liver donation including the MHV, the presence of a large segment VIII hepatic vein mandates division of the MHV proximal to the insertion of segment VIII hepatic vein for preservation of venous drainage of the right anterior sector.[18]

Hepatic angiography is not needed nowadays unless the hepatic artery anatomy is not clearly delineated by CT scan.

Magnetic resonance imaging is an excellent alternative to the CT scan, provided that expertise and high-quality equipment are available.

Delineation of the biliary tract before donor operation could be performed by CT or magnetic resonance imaging but both modalities could not replace operative cholangiography in terms of the exact delineation of segmental branches of the hepatic duct.

The indication for liver biopsy is for exclusion of fatty liver or pathology that endangers the donor after operation. Whether to perform liver biopsy or not as routine varies from centre to centre. Some centres advocate routine liver biopsy because a high incidence of steatosis is found among their potential donors,[19] while other centres relied on the BMI as an indicator for biopsy since obese people (BMI > 28) have a high incidence of steatosis.[20] In our centre, liver biopsy is performed only if there are signs of fatty liver on imaging. In our view, liver biopsy is an invasive procedure. Whether it should be done routinely or selectively depends on the prevalence of steatosis in the local population. The criteria of acceptance for donation in terms of the degree of fatty change also vary from centre to centre. We accept fatty liver up to 10%. Other centres accept a fatty liver graft up to 20% provided that the liver remnant to body weight ratio is more than 0.8%.[19] On this issue, Nadalin *et al.*[19] are very cautious. They recommended the donor should undergo dietary modification before reconsideration for donation if liver steatosis is 10–20% even if the remnant liver size is judged to be adequate.

As to the volumetry, the donor is accepted for right-liver donation if his/her left liver is ≥30% of the total liver volume[21] and his/her right liver is ≥40% of the estimated required liver weight of the recipient.[22]

Recipient Evaluation

The evaluation of recipients for LDLT should not differ from that of those accepted for DDLT. However, consideration should be given for anticipation of difficulty of recipient hepatectomy and graft implantation. Patients with multiple previous laparotomies and thrombosis of the portal or superior mesenteric vein are at a higher risk of massive bleeding and difficult implantation. A relatively small liver graft may not provide sufficient liver function to meet with the metabolic demand and the higher complication in such an instance. Retransplantations for portal vein thrombosis, hepatic artery thrombosis or biliary complications are probably less ideal cases for LDLT. On the other hand, patients with fulminant hepatic failure[23] or acute on chronic liver failure[24] are suitable candidates and the outcome is not different from those with cirrhosis.

Donor Left Hepatectomy

The abdomen is entered through a bilateral subcostal incision and a midline extension. Intraoperative ultrasonography is performed to study the anatomy of the MHV and the left hepatic vein. Doppler study is also performed to locate the site of hepatic artery for ease of localization after implantation. Cholecystectomy is then performed and the cystic duct cannulated for operative cholangiography. The location of the proposed division of the left hepatic duct is marked by a large size metal clip (Fig. 3). Excessive dissection of the left hepatic duct should not be done lest the hilar plate (and fine hepatic arterial branches running in it) is damaged. We advocate division of the left hepatic duct at the time of division of the liver parenchyma. To obtain complete filling of the intrahepatic duct by contrast, a bulldog vascular clamp is used to occlude the supraduodenal portion of the common bile duct temporarily. The sequence of filling of the intrahepatic ducts is observed on fluoroscopy. By this technique, accurate identification of the entire intrahepatic ducts, including the segment IV ducts could be obtained.

Hilar dissection is then conducted to free the left hepatic artery and left portal vein. In case the caudate lobe is included in the left-lobe graft, excessive dissection into the umbilical fissure must be avoided in order to

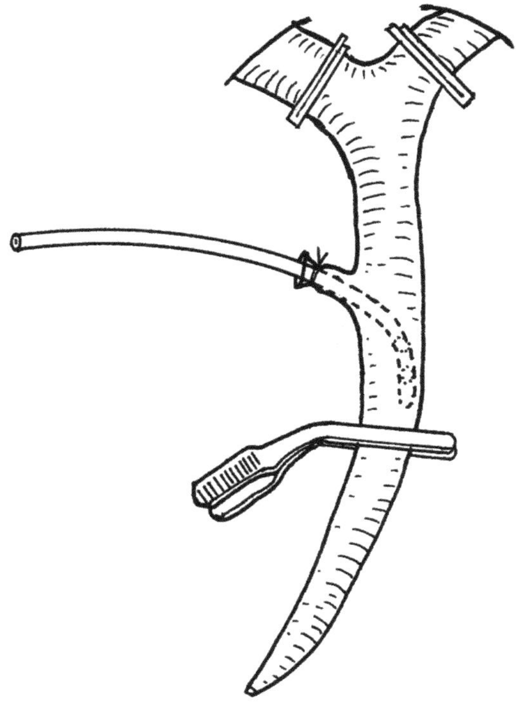

Figure 3: Diagram showing the procedure of operative cholangiogram obtained by cannulation of the cystic duct. The supraduodenal part of the common bile duct is temporarily occluded by a vascular clamp. A metal clip is used as a landmark for right or left hepatic duct division.

protect the arterial and portal vein supply to the caudate lobe. A large isolated caudate portal vein should be preserved for subsequent anastomosis.[25] The left lateral segment is then freed by dividing the lesser omentum and the left triangular ligament. If a large branch of the left hepatic artery arising from the left gastric artery is encountered, it must be preserved for subsequent reconstruction if needed. In case the caudate lobe is included in the graft, the left caudate is detached from the IVC and the ligamentum venosum is divided. The left and middle hepatic veins are encircled after the posterior surface of the caudate lobe is completely detached from the anterior surface of the IVC. A large caudate hepatic vein (5 mm) should be preserved for subsequent reconstruction.

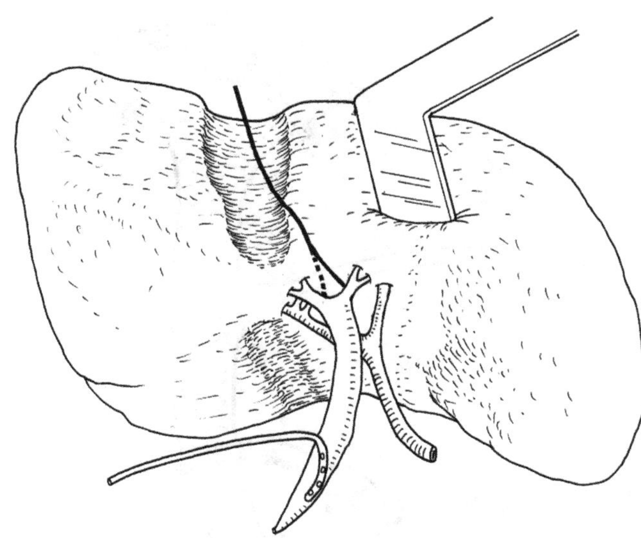

Figure 4: Diagram showing the inferior surface of the liver and the line of division of the liver parenchyma. For left-liver donor operation, the dividing line should reach the point of the proposed division site of left hepatic duct (solid line). For right-liver donor operation, the line should meet the point of right hepatic duct division (dotted line).

The Cantlie line is marked at the anterior surface of the liver by diathermy at a plane demarcated after temporary occlusion of the left hepatic artery and left portal vein. At the inferior surface of the liver, the division plane deviates to the left side of gallbladder fossa to meet the proposed dividing line of the left hepatic duct (Fig. 4). Division of the liver is made by ultrasonic dissector without inflow vascular occlusion. The MHV is encountered at the transection plane near to the liver hilum. At this point, the MHV trunk may be large if it originates from segment V. It is divided and transfixed. The liver transection should then proceed on the right side of the MHV which is preferably exposed all the way down to the junction with the IVC. The exposed MHV is used as a guide for the plane of liver transection. Under a low central venous pressure and complete muscle relaxation, bleeding during liver transection would not be excessive. The major site of bleeding comes from the MHV. If that occurs, temporary Pringle manoeuvre can be used to reduce the bleeding rate, accurate delineation of the site of bleeding and precise haemostasis.[26]

The role of inflow vascular occlusion in LDLT is controversial. The current practice of transplant surgeons varies from not using it at all to selective or routine use. The blood loss volume of our donor during hepatectomy without inflow vascular occlusion is about 200–400 ml. It is comparable with those series which employ Pringle manoeuvre routinely.[27] A prospective randomised trial is needed to show the advantage of routine Pringle manoeuvre in donor hepatectomy. However, in case the central venous pressure could not be brought down satisfactorily without affecting the blood pressure, Pringle manoeuvre would be a useful measure to reduce bleeding from the transection surface and expedite transection.

On approaching the liver hilum, we perform cholangiogram again, using the metal clip as an indicator for the site of proposed division of the left hepatic duct. After division of the left hepatic duct, the stump on the confluence side is closed by 6-0 PDS. Another cholangiogram is performed to ensure that the confluence is not damaged. After that, the liver parenchyma is divided vertically until the IVC is seen if the caudate lobe is included in the graft. Otherwise, the transection plane goes horizontally to the fissure in between the left caudate and the left lateral segment.

Harvesting of the left-liver graft starts with clamping of the left portal vein and left hepatic artery by vascular clamp and the middle and left hepatic vein by vascular stapler (TA* 30 V3 (2.5 mm), AutoSuture, Tyco Healthcare, Norwalk, CT, USA). The vessels are carefully divided and the graft is delivered to a basin containing ice sludges. Flushing of the left-liver graft is performed by putting a cannula into the left portal vein. The cannula is kept in place by pinching the portal vein in between the surgeon's left index finger and the thumb. Ligature is not employed as it will damage the portal vein wall. Currently, about 1.5 litres of HTK solution (Dr Frank Köhler, Chermie GmbH, Alsebach-Hähnlein, Germany) is used. The hepatic artery is also cannulated for short distance and flushing by about 50 ml HTK solution under gravity. After flushing, the graft is weighed. If the left and middle hepatic veins are separated, they are joined together in the form of venoplasty to facilitate implantation.[28]

In the donor, meticulous suturing of the left portal vein stump is made. Caution is exercised to avoid narrowing the right portal vein. The left hepatic artery is ligated. Doppler ultrasonography is performed to ensure patency of the portal vein and hepatic artery. Methylene blue is instilled into the biliary tract to look for bile leakage at the liver transection surface, hilar plate and hepatic duct stump. If seen, meticulous suturing is made. Abdominal drain is not required.

Recipient Hepatectomy and Left-Liver Graft Implantation

A generous bilateral subcostal incision and upward midline extension is made. The xiphoid process is routinely removed to allow approach to the suprahepatic IVC vertically. Hilar dissection is made to free the right and left hepatic artery, the common hepatic duct, the right and left portal vein and its main trunk. The tissue around the common hepatic duct is preserved as far as possible in order to retain its blood supply. It is divided close to the liver hilum so as to retain enough length for subsequent duct-to-duct anastomosis. For the division of the hepatic artery, the stump on the recipient side is controlled by an Acland microvascular clamp (S&T, Neuhausen, Switzerland) because it induces the least tissue trauma.[29] Simply ligating the stump may result in intimal dissection of the artery leading to the necessity of dissecting other arteries for anastomosis. The left and right portal vein must be free for the full length in the case of left-liver graft operation because not infrequently the left portal vein of the graft may not be long enough for tension-free anastomosis.

After hilar dissection, the right and left triangular ligaments are detached and the caudate hepatic vein branches are divided from the IVC. The portal vein is not divided until the separation of the IVC from the liver is completed and liver graft is available. Then, the main portal vein is clamped and the right and left portal veins divided close to the liver hilum. The right hepatic vein is clamped, divided and the stump is sutured. The middle and left hepatic veins are cross-clamped by Satinsky vascular clamp and divided, thus allowing delivery of the explant out of the abdominal cavity. The IVC is mobilised from the retroperitoneum. Several lumbar and phrenic veins may have to be ligated and divided before the IVC is completely mobilised from the diaphragm down to the level of right adrenal vein. After haemostasis of the retroperitoneum, the IVC is occluded by a cotton tape on the caudal side and a strong vascular clamp on the cephalad side (Fig. 5). The clamp controlling the middle and

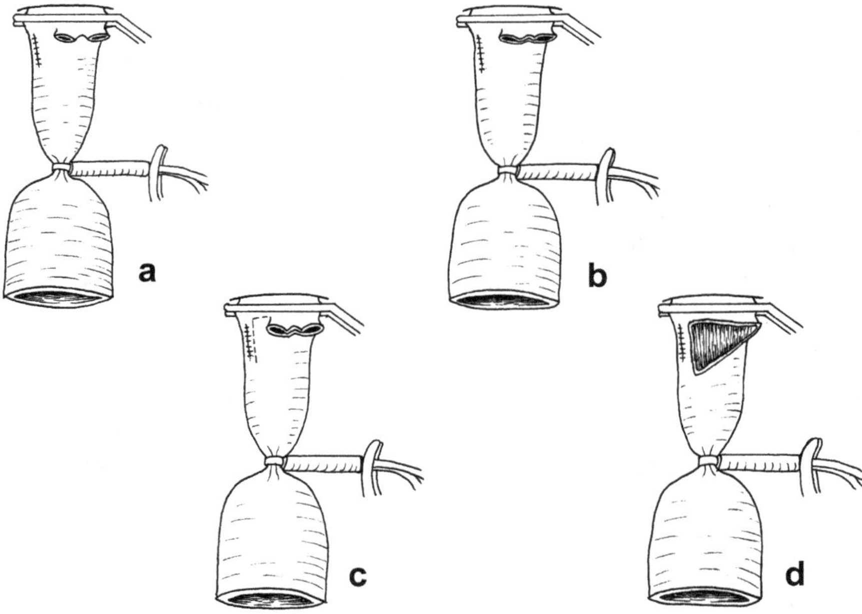

Figure 5: Diagram showing the creation of a large triangular opening in the recipient inferior vena cava for matching the size of the left-liver graft.

left hepatic veins is removed. The hepatic vein stump is slit open and cut into the anterior wall of the IVC to fashion a large triangular opening that matches in size with the hepatic vein opening of the left-liver graft. Redundant tissue of the hepatic vein wall is trimmed away to avoid folding-in of the anastomosis. The implantation starts with the hepatic vein anastomosis performed in a triangular fashion using 5-0 Prolene. Caudate hepatic vein anastomosis is performed if a large caudate vein is present by making a size-matched opening on the anterior wall of IVC. After the hepatic vein anastomosis is completed, the portal vein of the left-liver graft is inspected for correct orientation and clamped by a bulldog vascular clamp. The vascular clamp and tape controlling the IVC is then released to allow restoration of the IVC blood flow. At this time, the liver graft is partially perfused by blood regurgitating from the hepatic vein. Gradual re-warming of the graft will take place while the portal vein anastomosis is completed. To avoid redundancy, the length of the graft portal vein and recipient portal vein is adjusted and the ends trimmed if necessary. Portal vein anastomosis is performed by 6-0 Prolene. Hepatic artery anastomosis is performed by 9-0 nylon (Ethilon; Ethicos Inc, Somewille, NJ, USA) on a 9-0-gauge micropoint needle under operating microscope. Biliary reconstruction is by duct-to-duct anastomosis or hepatico-jejunostomy. Previously, hepatico-jejunostomy was thought to be the only reconstruction method for left-liver graft. Recently, more and more surgeons perform duct-to-duct anastomosis.[30] The latter procedure is more advantageous as contamination of the operative field by bowel flora could be avoided, the procedure is simpler and access to the biliary anastomosis could be obtained via endoscopic retrograde cholangiopancreatography. The decision to stent the biliary anastomosis is controversial. Currently, we do not insert a T-tube or stent in either duct-to-duct anastomosis[31] or hepatico-jejunostomy and observe no deleterious effect. In case the graft hepatic duct orifice is tiny and hepatico-jejunostomy is made, some surgeons advocate insertion of an external biliary stent to prevent partial occlusion of the anastomosis by swollen mucosa and subsequent cholangitis. However, the value of such approach has not been documented by prospective randomised trial. Before wound closure, careful inspection is made for bile leakage and complete haemostasis. The liver graft is fixed by suturing the falciform ligament to the anterior abdominal wall to prevent rotation into the right subphrenic cavity. The latter phenomenon may lead to graft congestion (as a result of MHV kinking[32]) or poor vascular inflow (as a result of folding of the portal vein) and ultimately graft failure. Doppler ultrasonography is therefore a 'must' procedure before and after wound closure to check the patency of the blood vessels. Finally, the wound is closed. Currently, we do not insert any abdominal drain.

Donor Right Hepatectomy

The initial step of right-liver donor hepatectomy is similar to that of left-liver donor hepatectomy. After cholecystectomy and cannulation of the cystic duct, the right-liver hilum is gently dissected to expose the right hepatic duct. A large size metal clip is applied to the liver capsule at the site of proposed division of the right hepatic duct (Fig. 3). 'Real-time' operative cholangiography is performed preferably with temporary occlusion of the supraduodenal portion of the common bile duct. Under the fluoroscopy, the right-posterior sector duct (being in the most dorsal position) will show up first, followed by the right-anterior sector duct, left hepatic duct, segment II and III ducts, and finally the segment IV duct (being in the most ventral position).[33] Minor branches arising from the right-posterior sector duct or left hepatic duct are usually the caudate branches (segments Ir and Il). They are sometimes thick and induce confusion in recognition of the anatomy. The segment Ir duct will most likely be encountered during transection of the caudate lobe. At the liver hilum, the segmental branches of the hepatic duct may overlap with each other and induce difficulty in identification. To produce a clear picture, counterclockwise rotation of the X-ray tube will produce an image free of overlapping because the transverse axis of the liver hilum is usually oblique in relation to the transverse axis of the donor's abdominal cavity.[33]

After the operative cholangiogram, dissection in the right-liver hilum will expose the right hepatic artery and right portal vein. Caution is exercised not to dissect into the space in between the right hepatic duct and right hepatic artery because there may be tiny (but important) arterial branches supplying the right hepatic duct. For the dissection of the right portal vein, a caudate lobe portal vein may have to be ligated and divided allowing sufficient length of the right portal vein for subsequent reconstruction. However, a large vein in this location may be the segment VI portal vein. If significant ischemia is induced by occluding the vein, such vein should not be sacrificed.

Temporary occlusion of the right hepatic artery and right portal vein will produce the demarcation between the right and left liver. The transection plane should be based on this demarcation line. At the inferior surface of the liver, the division line is deviated to the left side of the gallbladder fossa to meet the point of the proposed division of the right hepatic duct (Fig. 4). With such design, liver tissue are left covering the right hepatic duct ensuring that the right hepatic duct is not denuded during liver transection. Division of the liver is made by ultrasonic dissector without inflow vascular occlusion. At the transection plane near to the liver hilum the segment IV hepatic vein flowing into the MHV will be encountered. It should be divided and sutured. Subsequently the MHV will be exposed on the left side and used as the guidance plane for liver transection until the root of the MHV is reached. The junction of the MHV is gently separated from the segment IVb hepatic vein and the left hepatic vein. The tissue at the back of the MHV is also trimmed away by the ultrasonic dissector if it is thick. The caudate lobe is divided by ultrasonic dissector until the entire IVC is exposed. Lifting up the caudate lobe by a pair of right-angle instrument will expedite the transection.

The need for inclusion of the MHV in the right-liver graft is controversial. We consider that inclusion is necessary because it is the major drainage vein of segments V and VIII. By multivariate analysis, occlusion of the MHV is one of the independent significant factors affecting hospital mortality of the recipient.[34] Several centres did not find inclusion of the MHV necessary. However, these centres utilise right-liver grafts, which are always above 0.8% of body weight, and the recipients have a relatively low MELD score.[35] A large-liver graft may compensate for the relative lack of venous outflow in the right anterior sector and in the absence of severe portal hypertension, small-for-size graft injury may be less severe. On the other hand, our patients had high MELD score (median 27) before transplant and 28% of the liver grafts are smaller than 0.8% of the body weight. With routine inclusion of the MHV, a smaller graft could be used and the clinical application could be much widened. Other centres adopt a more flexible approach.[36] They would include the MHV in the graft if the donor-to-recipient body weight ratio is less than one, right lobe-to-recipient body weight ratio <50% and there are multiple small segment V and VIII hepatic veins.

The right hepatic duct is usually divided at the time of liver transection. We prefer to perform another cholangiogram to ensure that the division site is exact and two or more ductal openings are avoided. The right hepatic duct is divided by a pair of scissors. Brisk bleeding is usually encountered during the duct division. The bleeding site should be sutured immediately to avoid unnecessary blood loss.

The graft retrieval starts with clamping and dividing the right portal vein and right hepatic artery. The middle and right hepatic veins are occluded by vascular staplers and divided on the graft side. The graft is then delivered to an ice-sludge basin. HTK solution is used to flush the portal vein. The hepatic artery is also flushed for 50 ml.

The middle and right hepatic veins of the right-liver graft are joined together to form a large triangular opening.[37] The procedure starts with pulling together the two veins at the appropriate sites using 6-0 Prolene sutures. The newly created septum is then divided vertically and sutured horizontally. The base of the triangular opening (along the axis of the IVC groove) and the height (perpendicular to the base) are measured. The graft is then weighed and put into the sterile bag and immersed in an ice chamber.

In the donor, the portal vein stump is carefully sutured to avoid purse-string effect on the main trunk. Fine suture and closely spaced suturing should be used and the knot should be tied before the vascular clamp is removed. The right hepatic artery stump is ligated twice. Methylene blue is instilled into the biliary tract for checking bile leakage. Bile leakage may occur from the right hepatic duct stump, caudate braches, hilar plate or the liver transection surface. If found, meticulous suturing must be made. Finally the cystic cannula is removed and the cystic duct ligated by absorbable material. The abdominal wall is closed without drainage.[38]

Recipient Hepatectomy and Right-Liver Graft Implantation

The recipient hepatectomy of right-liver graft recipient is not different from those of left-liver. The right and left hepatic arteries are dissected near to the liver hilum to preserve maximum length for subsequent implantation. The right hepatic artery is usually located on the right side and underneath the common hepatic duct. To protect the blood supply of the common hepatic duct arising from the right hepatic artery, the right hepatic artery should not be mobilised from the common bile duct. There is usually a long length of right hepatic artery at the right liver hilum to be freed and preserved for subsequent anastomosis. The common hepatic duct is divided close to the liver hilum. It is not necessary and probably inadvisable to dissect and divide the common hepatic duct in the hilar plate since it is unusual to require a long length of common hepatic duct for duct-to-duct anastomosis and dividing it in the hilar plate may result in dividing the unrecognised caudate branches. Missing these branches may be the cause of postoperative bile leakage. For the dissection of the portal vein, unlike the left-liver operation, it is not necessary to free the full length of the right and left portal veins because we found anastomosis of the graft right portal vein to the recipient main portal vein preferable and successful.

The diseased liver is then mobilised from the IVC in a similar manner as in the left-liver operation. When the liver graft is available, the portal vein is occluded and divided, then, the right hepatic vein is clamped and divided while the common trunk of the middle and left hepatic veins is clamped, divided and sutured.

The IVC is cross-clamped by a vascular clamp and cotton tape (Fig. 6). A triangular opening is made by slitting open the right hepatic vein and cutting into the anterior wall of the IVC. Redundant tissues are

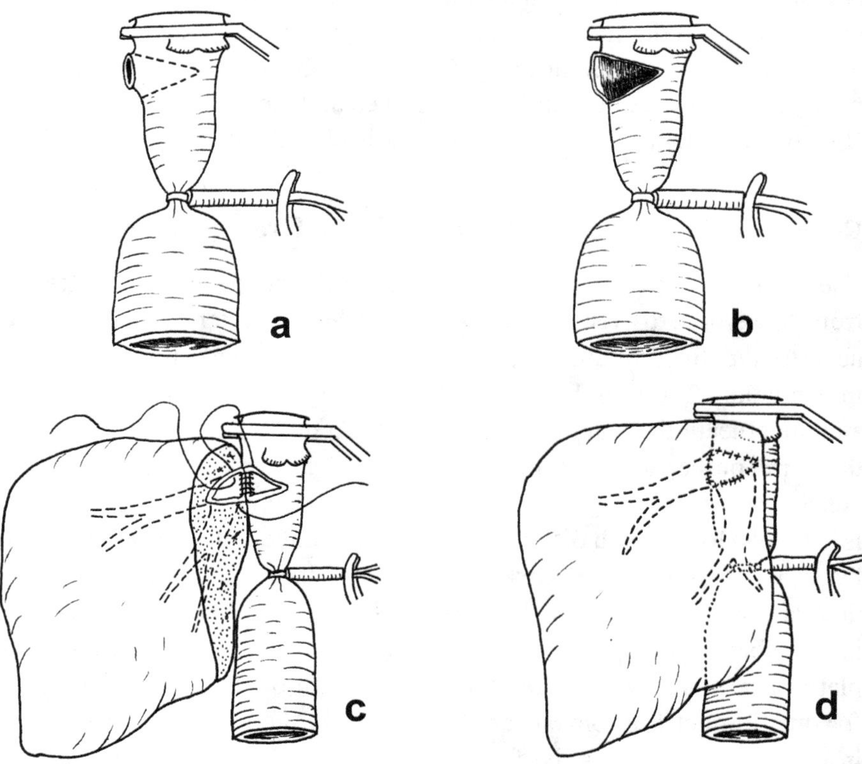

Figure 6: Diagram showing the creation of a large triangular opening in the recipient inferior vena cava for anastomosing to the donor right-liver graft.

removed and a triangular opening similar in size to the orifice of the hepatic vein of the liver graft is made. Implantation is then made by 5-0 Prolene sutures made on three sides of the triangle. On complete suturing, the knot is tied with a growth factor of 5 mm to avoid purse-string effect of the suturing. Additional hepatic vein anastomosis is made if inferior or middle-right hepatic vein is present in the graft. After the portal vein is controlled the IVC clamp is released to allow restoration of the blood flow. The graft right portal vein is anastomosed to the recipient main portal vein. Careful adjustment is made to avoid redundancy. The effect of redundancy will become obvious when the graft regenerates and rotates to the left side of the abdominal cavity. It is a possible cause of portal vein thrombosis.

Hepatic artery is reconstructed by 9-0 nylon suture under an operating microscope. Not infrequently the left hepatic artery of the recipient is used for anastomosis since it results in a straighter course than that using the right hepatic artery.

Biliary reconstruction is performed by duct-to-duct anastomosis in most of the instances. In about 30% of the instances, two ductal openings are present. If they are near to each other, ductoplasty can be performed to join them together to form a single orifice. In case of two or more hepatic orifices that are at a large distance from each other, hepaticojejunostomy is preferred.

After complete haemostasis, the abdominal cavity is thoroughly washed by normal saline. The abdominal wound is closed without drainage.

What has been described above is our current technique. The major difference from that used in other centres is the inclusion of the MHV in the graft. In case the MHV is not included in the graft, but the segments V and VIII hepatic veins are sizeable (>5 mm), many surgeons advocate restoration of draining the right-anterior sector by jump graft[39–43] to relieve graft congestion. The material used included saphenous vein, superficial femoral vein, recipient left portal vein and cryopreserved iliac vein.

Postoperative Care of the Donor

The donor is cared for in the intensive care unit on the first postoperative day. Adequate pain relief is achieved by patient-controlled analgesia.

Chest physiotherapy is mandatory. They are also given incentive spirometry to expedite recovery of the respiratory function. H_2-antagonist is routinely prescribed but we have changed it to proton pump inhibitor recently. It is given for four weeks. Systematic antibiotic (Augmentin, GlaxoSmithKline, Brentford, Middlesex, UK) is given for two doses only. The donor is given oral fluid as soon as the bowel function returns. Before resumption of oral feeding, intravenous fluid administration is restricted unless obvious hypovolemia is seen. Excessive fluid administration is harmful as it raises the central venous pressure and impedes the venous drainage of the liver remnant. On the other hand, if the donor requires excessive amount of fluid to maintain blood pressure, that may signify that the liver function is suboptimal. Prompt administration of inotrope must be made before the donor is overloaded by intravenous fluid.

Postoperative Management of the Recipient

The recipient is nursed in the intensive care unit until his or her condition is stable. Fluid administration is restricted. Usually no fluid other than concentrated albumin solution is given immediately after the operation unless obvious hypovolemia is seen. Since the patient usually retains much fluid before and during the transplant operation and when the liver function improves, fluid accumulated in the extravascular compartment returning into the circulation will predispose him or her to pulmonary edema. However, the liver function in the first postoperative two to three days may be suboptimal. Inotropes is therefore routinely given until the blood pressure is well maintained and urine output is satisfactory.

In the early postoperative period the international normalized ratio may be high. Fresh frozen plasma is not routinely given unless the international normalized ratio is above 2.5. Likewise, platelet concentrates are not given unless procedures that are at high risk of bleeding are performed.

As the patient is frequently immunocompromised, the incidence of catheter infection is quite high. To prevent catheter infection, pulmonary artery catheter and central venous catheters are removed on the next postoperative day unless the condition of the patient is unstable.

Systemic antibiotic is given for less than three days unless the patient has evidence of sepsis preoperatively. Topical application of mupirocin cream to the nasal orifice and groin creases and axillae is given to prevent methicillin-resistant staphylococcus aureus (MRSA) infection. Previously, one dose of rifampicin was given to our patients at the time of surgery to prevent MRSA infection.[23] Since the MRSA infection rate is low in our recent patients and rifampicin may interact with FK506, rifampicin is no longer given to the recipients. The high MRSA infection rate in the past might be related to suboptimal graft function. With improvement of surgical technique and satisfactory graft function, anti-MRSA coverage may not be necessary. Fluconazole is routinely given. For patients who have haemodialysis before transplant and those with positive fungal culture in the urine, intravenous liposomal amphotericin B (Ambisome, Gilead Sciences, Foster City, CA, USA) is advisable.

Systemic heparin administration or agents to reduce coagulation are not needed for prevention of hepatic artery thrombosis. However, daily Doppler ultrasonography is advisable to detect early hepatic artery thrombosis especially when the arterial anastomosis is thought to be precarious.

Donor Complications and Outcome

Despite the fact that donors are healthy persons and operations are performed on normal livers, donor complications do occur. Using Clavien[44] complication classification, the incidences of grade I, II, III complications among our first 200 right-liver live donors are 13.5%, 4% and 4%, respectively. The overall complication rate is 21.5%. The complication rate decreased from 34% in our first 50 liver donors to 16% in our second 50 right-liver donors but remained at 16% in the third and fourth 50 donors. The majority of the complications were minor wound infections. The others included pressure sores, urinary tract infection, pleural effusion, bile duct stenosis, and haemoperitoneum. Bile leakage has not occurred in our donors. We ascribe it to meticulous ligation and clipping of all branches during liver transection and avoidance of excessive tissue coagulation. Life-threatening complications (Clavien grade III) and hospital mortality (Clavien grade IV) have not occurred in our donors but one donor died of duodenal ulcer perforated into the IVC (duodenocaval fistula) ten weeks after the right-liver donation. The duodenal ulcer had been asymptomatic before the acute presentation. The donor had been given

H_2-antagonist for two weeks after the operation. Since the occurrence of the complications, we now cover the donors with a four-week course of proton-pump inhibitor after the operation.

More serious complications have happened in other series. Donors lapsing into liver failure and listing for liver transplantation or receiving liver transplantation have been reported.[45]

Early or hospital mortalities of donors did occur in several liver transplant centres.[45–53] The estimated donor mortality rate is 0.5%. The incidence is higher than in kidney live-donor operations. The causes of death include pulmonary embolism, pulmonary infection due to uncommon pathogen, emphysematous gastritis, liver failure due to congenital lipodystrophy and non-alcoholic steatohepatitis, acute pancreatitis and cerebral haemorrhage. Donor suicide was also reported.[45] The majority of causes of donor death appeared not to be related to the operation itself. However, the surgeon should not be excused because some of these complications arose from deficiency in selection of donors and perioperative care. It is fair to state that complications and mortality are to be expected for an ultra-major operation, but transplant surgeons should exercise utmost care and diligence to avoid complications in future donors.

Recipient Outcome

At our centre, the hospital mortality of the first 200 right-liver LDLT is 5.4%. With increasing experience and modification of technique, the median intensive care unit stay duration has decreased from 15 days to two days and blood transfusion requirement from 11 units to two units. About 20% of recipients operated in the last four years did not require exogenous blood transfusion. The hospital mortality is about the same for patients with cirrhosis (4.7%), acute on chronic liver failure (6.8%) and fulminant hepatic failure (5.9%), despite a major difference in their MELD scores (16, 36 and 36, respectively).

We perform fewer left-liver LDLT than right-liver LDLT. There have been three hospital mortalities out of 16 recipients (18.5%). All the survivors have remained well since the operation. In Japan, where most left-liver LDLT are performed, the graft survival rate is about 85%.

The long-term survival rate of right-liver LDLT is improving. In our centre, the five-year survival rate has improved from 70% in the first 50 cases to 85% in the second 100 cases. The long-term survival rate of right-liver LDLT is similar to that of DDLT despite a smaller liver graft and a more complex operation. However, in the USA, LDLT was reported to have a lower survival rate than DDLT.[54,55]

The major long-term complication of the recipient remains to be stenosis of biliary anastomosis. It is not known whether the anastomosis stenotic rate could be influenced by the type of anastomosis (hepaticojejunostomy vs duct-to-duct anastomosis) or use of stent across the anastomosis. A prospective randomised study has not been conducted in LDLT. Extrapolating the results of studies of T-tube stenting of bile duct in DDLT, we speculate that the use of stent would not produce any incremental benefit. However, we admit that without stenting, late stenosis of bile duct did occur in our patients. The incidence of late biliary stenosis is about 20%, which, however, is similar to many reported series in which routine stenting is performed.

Impact of LDLT

The innovation of LDLT has obviously solved the problem of organ shortage, especially in countries where deceased donor organ donation is scarce or prohibited. The impact is more obvious with the use of right-liver LDLT as the operation allows a smaller donor to donate the right liver to a larger size recipient. With right-liver LDLT, patients waiting for DDLT[24] and those with acute liver failure benefit.[23] Their waiting time is much shortened, transplant rate increased and survival rate increased.

However, LDLT has been reported to have a higher incidence of hepatitis C virus and hepatocellular carcinoma (HCC) recurrence.[54] For hepatitis C virus, a recent analysis showed that the survival outcome is not different from that of DDLT.[56,57] The unsatisfactory result in the early series could be due to technical errors. For HCC, the higher recurrence rate is probably real. In our centre, the recurrence rate of HCC after LDLT is 16%, whereas that of DDLT is 0% ($P < 0.05$). It is postulated that the higher regeneration rate and reperfusion injury of small grafts in LDLT provides an environment favorable for HCC cell implantation and growth in the graft. It is also possible that in LDLT, for preservation of the IVC, more liver manipulation is required, leading to tumour compression and cancer cell dissemination. However, it is not unlikely that patients who have received DDLT are the highly selected patients because only those with slowly growing HCC who could wait for deceased donor grafts could receive the transplantation. The cancer cell behaviour may be different for these two groups. Further studies on patient selection criteria and innovation of surgical technique are required to improve long-term outcome of LDLT for HCC.

Future perspective

To maintain LDLT as a viable option, liver transplant centres have to reduce donor morbidity to less than 20% and mortality rate to less than 0.5%. Whether the mortality rate could be eliminated entirely is questionable. Given the ultra-major nature of the operation, mortality due to uncommon conditions will occur. The transplant community has to accept mortality, albeit undesirable, for the salvage of many patients with terminal liver failure. LDLT will continue in practice until ample supply of deceased organs is available. Before that occurs, further technical refinement is required to improve the results, particularly in biliary anastomosis and HCC patients.

References

1. Raia S, Nery JR, Mies S. Liver transplantation from live donors. *Lancet* 1989;2:497.
2. Couinaud C. Liver anatomy: portal (and suprahepatic) or biliary segmentation. *Dig. Surg.* 1999;16:459–67.
3. Strong RW, Lynch SV, Ong TH, Matsunami H, Koido Y, Balderson GA. Successful liver transplantation from a living donor to her son. *N. Engl. J. Med.* 1990;322:1505–7.
4. Haberal M, Bilgin N, Velidedeoglu E, Turan M. Living-donor organ transplantation at our centre. *Transplant. Proc.* 1993;25:3147–8.

5. Ichida T, Matsunami H, Kawasaki S, Makuuchi M, Harada T, Itoh S, Asakura H. Living related-donor liver transplantation from adult to adult for primary biliary cirrhosis. *Ann. Intern. Med.* 1995;122:275–6.
6. Lo CM, Gertsch P, Fan ST. Living unrelated liver transplantation between spouses for fulminant hepatic failure. *Br. J. Surg.* 1995;82:1037.
7. Urata K, Kawasaki S, Matsunami H, Hashikura Y, Ikegami T, Ishizone S, Momose Y, Komiyama A, Makuuchi M. Calculation of child and adult standard liver volume for liver transplantation. *Hepatology* 1995;21:1317–21.
8. Takayama T, Makuuchi M, Kubota K, Sano K, Harihara Y, Kawarasaki H. Living related transplantation of left liver plus caudate lobe. *J. Am. Coll. Surg.* 2000;190:635–8.
9. Miyagawa S, Hashikura Y, Miwa S, Ikegami T, Urata K, Terada M, Kubota T, Nakata T, Kawasaki S. Concomitant caudate lobe resection as an option for donor hepatectomy in adult living related liver transplantation. *Transplantation* 1998; 66:661–3.
10. Inomoto T, Nishizawa F, Sasaki H, Terajima H, Shirakata Y, Miyamoto S, Nagata I, Fujimoto M, Moriyasu F, Tanaka K, Yamaoka Y. Experiences of 120 microsurgical reconstructions of hepatic artery in living related liver transplantation. *Surgery* 1996;119:20–6.
11. Lo CM, Fan ST, Liu CL, Lo RJ, Lau GK, Wei WI, Li JH, Ng IO, Wong J. Extending the limit on the size of adult recipient in living-donor liver transplantation using extended right lobe graft. *Transplantation* 1997;63:1524–8.
12. Kiuchi T, Inomata Y, Uemoto S, Satomura K, Egawa H, Okajima H, Yamaoka Y, Tanaka K. A hepatic graft tuberculosis transmitted from a living related donor. *Transplantation* 1997;63:905–7.
13. Durand F, Ettorre GM, Douard R, Denninger MH, Kianmanesh A, Sommacale D, Farges O, Valla D, Belghiti J. Donor safety in living related liver transplantation: underestimation of the risks for deep vein thrombosis and pulmonary embolism. *Liver Transpl.* 2002;8:118–20.
14. Merten GJ, Burgess WP, Gray LV, Holleman JH, Roush TS, Kowalchuk GJ, Bersin RM, Van Moore A, Simonton CA 3rd, Rittase RA, Norton HJ, Kennedy TP. Prevention of contrast-induced nephropathy with sodium bicarbonate: a randomized controlled trial. *JAMA* 2004;291:2328–34.
15. Ikegami T, Kawasaki S, Matsunami H, Hashikura Y, Nakazawa Y, Miyagawa S, Furuta S, Iwanaka T, Makuuchi M. Should all hepatic arterial branches be constructed in living related liver transplantation? *Surgery* 1996;119:431–6.

16. Fan ST, Lo CM, Liu CL, Wang WX, Wong J. Safety and necessity of including the middle hepatic vein in the right lobe graft in adult-to-adult live-donor liver transplantation. *Ann. Surg.* 2003;238:137–48.
17. Chan SC, Lo CM, Liu CL, Wong Y, Fan ST, Wong J. Tailoring donor hepatectomy per segment IV venous drainage in right-lobe live-donor liver transplantation. *Liver Transpl.* 2004;10:755–62.
18. Kishi Y, Sugawara Y, Akamatsu N, Kaneko J, Matsui Y, Kokudo N, Makuuchi M. Sharing the middle hepatic vein between donor and recipient: left-liver graft procurement preserving a large segment VIII branch in donor. *Liver Transpl.* 2004;10:1208–12.
19. Nadalin S, Malago M, Valentin-Gamazo C, Testa G, Baba HA, Liu C, Fruhauf NR, Schaffer R, Gerken G, Frilling A, Broelsch CE. Preoperative donor liver biopsy for adult living-donor liver transplantation: risks and benefits. *Liver Transpl.* 2005;11:980–6.
20. Rinella ME, Alonso E, Rao S, Whitington P, Fryer J, Abecassis M, Superina R, Flamm SL, Blei AT. Body mass index as a predictor of hepatic steatosis in living liver donors. *Liver Transpl.* 2001;7:409–14.
21. Fan ST, Lo CM, Liu CL, Yong BH, Chan JK, Ng IO. Safety of donors in live-donor liver transplantation using right-lobe grafts. *Arch. Surg.* 2000; 135:336–40.
22. Lo CM, Fan ST, Liu CL, Wei WI, Lo RJ, Lai CL, Chan JK, Ng IO, Fung A, Wong J. Adult-to-adult living-donor liver transplantation using extended right-lobe grafts. *Ann. Surg.* 1997;226:261–9.
23. Liu CL, Fan ST, Lo CM, Yong BH, Fung AS, Wong J. Right-lobe live-donor liver transplantation improves survival of patients with acute liver failure. *Br. J. Surg.* 2002;89:317–22.
24. Liu CL, Lam B, Lo CM, Fan ST. Impact of right-lobe live-donor liver transplantation on patients waiting for liver transplantation. *Liver Transpl.* 2003; 9:863–9.
25. Kokudo N, Sugawara Y, Kaneko J, Imamura H, Sano K, Makuuchi M. Reconstruction of isolated caudate portal vein in left-liver graft. *Liver Transpl.* 2004;10:1163–5.
26. Man K, Fan ST, Ng IO, Lo CM, Liu CL, Wong J. Prospective evaluation of Pringle manoeuver in hepatectomy for liver tumours by a randomized study. *Ann. Surg.* 1997;226:704–11.

27. Imamura H, Takayama T, Sugawara Y, Kokudo N, Aoki, Kaneko J, Matsuyama Y, Sano K, Maema A, Makuuchi M. Pringle's manoeuvre in living donors. *Lancet* 2002;360:2049–50.
28. de Villa VH, Chen CL, Chen YS, Wang CC, Wang SH, Chiang YC, Cheng YF, Huang TL, Jawan B, Cheung HK. Outflow tract reconstruction in living-donor liver transplantation. *Transplantation* 2000;70:1604–8.
29. Wei WI, Lam LK, Ng RW, Liu CL, Lo CM, Fan ST, Wong J. Microvascular reconstruction of the hepatic artery in live-donor liver transplantation: experience across a decade. *Arch. Surg.* 2004;139:304–7.
30. Soejima Y, Shimada M, Suehiro T, Kishikawa K, Minagawa R, Hiroshige S, Ninomiya M, Shiotani S, Harada N, Sugimachi K. Feasibility of duct-to-duct biliary reconstruction in left-lobe adult-living-donor liver transplantation. *Transplantation* 2003;75:557–9.
31. Liu CL, Lo CM, Chan SC, Fan ST. Safety of duct-to-duct biliary reconstruction in right-lobe live-donor liver transplantation without biliary drainage. *Transplantation* 2004;77:726–32.
32. Poon RTP, Chan J, Fan ST. Left hepatic vein kinking after right trisegmentectomy: a potential cause of postoperative liver failure. *Hepatogastroenterology* 1998;45:508–9.
33. Fan ST, Lo CM, Liu CL, Tso WK, Wong J. Biliary reconstruction and complications of right-lobe live-donor liver transplantation. *Ann. Surg.* 2002;236:676–83.
34. Fan ST, Lo CM, Liu CL, Yong BH, Wong J. Determinants of hospital mortality of adult recipients of right-lobe live-donor liver transplantation. *Ann. Surg.* 2003;238:864–9.
35. Maluf DG, Stravitz RT, Cotterell AH, Posner MP, Nakatsuka M, Sterling RK, Luketic VA, Shiffman ML, Ham JM, Marcos A, Behnke MK, Fisher RA. Adult living donor versus deceased donor liver transplantation: a six-year single centre experience. *Am. J. Transplant.* 2005;5:149–56.
36. de Villa VH, Chen CL, Chen YS, Wang CC, Lin CC, Cheng YF, Huang TL, Jawan B, Eng HL. Right-lobe living-donor liver transplantation — addressing the middle hepatic vein controversy. *Ann. Surg.* 2003; 238:275–82.
37. Liu CL, Zhao Y, Lo CM, Fan ST. Hepatic venoplasty in right-lobe live-donor liver transplantation. *Liver Transpl.* 2003;9:1265–72.

38. Liu CL, Fan ST, Lo CM, Chan SC, Yong BH, Wong J. Safety of donor right hepatectomy without abdominal drainage: a prospective evaluation in 100 consecutive liver donors. *Liver Transpl.* 2005;11:314–9.
39. Sugawara Y, Makuuchi M, Akamatsu N, Kishi Y, Niiya T, Kaneko J, Imamura H, Kokudo N. Refinement of venous reconstruction using cryopreserved veins in right-liver grafts. *Liver Transpl.* 2004;10:541–7.
40. Lee SG, Lee YJ, Park KM, *et al.* Anterior segment congestion of a right-lobe graft in living-donor liver transplantation and its strategy to prevent congestion [in Korean]. *J. Korean Soc. Transpl.* 1999;13:213–8.
41. Sugawara Y, Makuuchi M, Sano K, Imamura H, Kaneko J, Ohkubo T, Matsui Y, Kokudo N. Vein reconstruction in modified right-liver graft for living-donor liver transplantation. *Ann. Surg.* 2003;237:180–5.
42. Kornberg A, Heyne J, Schotte U, Hommann M, Scheele J. Hepatic venous outflow reconstruction in right-lobe living-donor liver graft using recipient's superficial femoral vein. *Am. J. Transplant.* 2003;3:1444–7.
43. Dong G, Sankary HN, Malago M, Oberholzer J, Panaro F, Knight PS, Jarzembowski TM, Benedetti E, Testa G. Cadaver iliac vein outflow reconstruction in living-donor right-lobe liver transplantation. *J. Am. Coll. Surg.* 2004;199:504–7.
44. Dindo D, Demartines N, Clavien PA. Classification of surgical complications: a new proposal with evaluation in a cohort of 6,336 patients and results of a survey. *Ann. Surg.* 2004;240:205–13.
45. Brown RS, Jr, Russo MW, Lai M, Shiffman ML, Richardson MC, Everhart JE, Hoofnagle JH. A survey of liver transplantation from living adult donors in the United States. *N. Engl. J. Med.* 2003;348:818–25.
46. Boillot O, Dawahra M, Mechet I, Poncet G, Choucair A, Henry L, Boucaud C, Sagnard P, Scoazec JY. Liver transplantation using a right-liver lobe from a living donor. *Transplant. Proc.* 2002;34:773–6.
47. Malago M, Testa G, Frilling A, Nadalin S, Valentin-Gamazo C, Paul A, Lang H, Treichel U, Cicinnati V, Gerken G, Broelsch CE. Right living-donor liver transplantation: an option for adult patients: single institution experience with 74 patients. *Ann. Surg.* 2003;238:853–62.
48. Miller C, Florman S, Kim-Schluger L, Lento P, De La Garza J, Wu J, Xie B, Zhang W, Bottone E, Zhang D, Schwartz M. Fulminant and fatal gas gangrene of the stomach in a healthy live liver donor. *Liver Transpl.* 2004;10:1315–9.

49. Wiederkehr JC, Pereira JC, Ekermann M, Porto F, Kondo W, Nagima I, Amaral W, Camargo CA, Moreira M. Results of 132 hepatectomies for living-donor liver transplantation: report of one death. *Transplant. Proc.* 2005;37:1079–80.
50. Akabayashi A, Slingsby BT, Fujita M. The first donor death after living related liver transplantation in Japan. *Transplantation* 2004;77:634.
51. Broering DC, Wilms C, Bok P, Fischer L, Mueller L, Hillert C, Lenk C, Kim JS, Sterneck M, Schulz KH, Krupski G, Nierhaus A, Ameis D, Burdelski M, Rogiers X. Evolution of donor morbidity in living related liver transplantation: a single-centre analysis of 165 cases. *Ann. Surg.* 2004;240:1013–24.
52. Malago M, Rogiers X, Burdelski M, Broelsch CE. Living related liver transplantation: 36 cases at the University of Hamburg. *Transplant. Proc.* 1994; 26:3620–1.
53. Why did the transplant donor die? *The Times of India.* 12 July 2003.
54. Thuluvath PJ, Yoo HY. Graft and patient survival after adult live-donor liver transplantation compared to a matched cohort who received a deceased-donor transplantation. *Liver Transpl.* 2004;10:1263–8.
55. Abt PL, Mange KC, Olthoff KM, Markmann JF, Reddy KR, Shaked A. Allograft survival following adult-to-adult living-donor liver transplantation. *Am. J. Transplant.* 2004;4:1302–7.
56. Guo L, Orrego M, Rodriguez-Luna H, Balan V, Byrne T, Chopra K, Douglas DD, Harrison E, Moss A, Reddy KS, Williams JW, Rakela J, Mulligan D, Vargas HE. Living donor liver transplantation for hepatitis C-related cirrhosis: no difference in histological recurrence when compared to deceased donor liver transplantation recipients. *Liver Transpl.* 2006;12:560–5.
57. Schmeding M, Neumann UP, Puhl G, Bahra M, Neuhaus R, Neuhaus P. Hepatitis C recurrence and fibrosis progression are not increased after living donor liver transplantation: a single center study of 289 patients. *Liver Transpl.* 2007;13:687–92.

Chapter 4

Living Donor Pancreas Transplantation

David Sutherland, John Najarian and Rainer Gruessner

Introduction

Historically, the pancreas was the first extrarenal organ that was transplanted successfully from a living donor (LD),[1] done as a segmental graft (distal pancreas – body and tail) from a mother to her diabetic daughter at the University of Minnesota Hospital on 20 June 1979, restoring insulin-independence,[2] the objective of the procedure. An earlier attempt at an extrarenal LD transplant – of a small bowel segment – by Ralph Deterling in Boston in 1964 was not successful because the recipient died within 12 hours.[3]

The first LD segmental pancreas transplant was done 11 and a half years after the world's first deceased donor pancreas transplant (also segmental), also done at the University of Minnesota by Kelly and Lillehei *et al.*[4] in December 1966. In the interval between the first deceased- and first living-donor pancreas transplants, (1) a series of 13 more deceased-donor pancreas transplants (all whole organ; only one functioned >1 year, the others failed from either technical complications related to the duodenum or from rejection) were done by Lillehei *et al.*[5] at the University of Minnesota, with the last in 1973[6]; (2) pancreas transplant programmes began at a few other centres[7] in the USA[8,9] and Europe[10,11] mainly using deceased-donor segmental grafts[9–11]; (3) a clinical islet transplant programme began in 1974 at the University of Minnesota[12,13] initially and mainly from deceased but with two from LDs[1,14] in the hope that a minimally invasive approach could replace solid organ pancreas transplantation for beta-cell replacement therapy in diabetes (it has not yet, but the islet programme continues to this day[15]); and (4) deceased-donor pancreas transplants (initially with segmental grafts) were resumed at the University of Minnesota in 1978,[16] a programme that also continues to this day.[17]

Thus, even though the first LD solid organ pancreas (segmental) transplant was done in 1979, this seminal event was preceded by two LD islet allografts done 21 and 11 months earlier in a pair of diabetic recipients, the islets being isolated from the distal (body and tail) pancreas excised in a manner identical to that done in the first LD segmental pancreas transplant case.[1] The rationale to do LD islet allografts was based on the unsatisfactory results with our initial deceased-donor islet allografts – only transient reduction in insulin requirements or a temporary period of C-peptide presence[13,14] – while at the same time our first islet autograft in early 1977 (preceding the first LD islet allograft by six months) preserved insulin-independence after a total pancreastectomy for chronic pancreatitis, an outcome duplicated in another patient five months before our second LD islet allograft.[14] In the late 1970s it was not clear whether the failure to ameliorate diabetes in recipients of deceased-donor islets was due to technical problems (inadequate organ preservation prior to or injury during isolation) or for immunological reasons. However, the successful islet autografts led us to believe that the technical problems could be overcome if rejection could be prevented.[14] Autologous islets were isolated immediately after pancreastectomy, eliminating prolonged pre-isolation preservation as a factor in outcome, and the use of a LD hemi-pancreas for islet allotransplantation did the same. Islet autografts could not be rejected, a situation that could only be duplicated with an isograft. However, even though the possibility of rejection of allogenic islets was not eliminated by using LDs, we knew from our experience with renal allografts that the incidence of rejection episodes or losses was lower in organs that came from living than from deceased donors.[18] Thus we thought that LD islet allografts had a reasonable probability of succeeding and that we would gain an understanding of the causes of failure of islet allografts from deceased donors.[1] The first LD islet transplant was done on 27 September 1977, the second on 12 July 1978,[1] just before pancreas transplants were restarted at the University of Minnesota on

25 July 1978.[16] The latter ended a five-year hiatus in pancreas transplantation at our institution since the last case in the Lillehei series.[5,6]

The courses of the two recipients of LD islets were described in detail in 1980 in a paper in *Diabetes* on a series of islet allografts and autografts at the University of Minnesota presented at a Kroc Foundation Conference in 1979.[14] The paper in *Diabetes*[14] focused on our initial islet autografts (three cases) and our second series of islet allografts, eight transplants in seven patients, since the initial series of ten deceased-donor islet transplants in another seven recipients had been described in detail previously.[13] In the *Diabetes* article[14] the two islet allografts from LDs were identified as Patient Nos 3 and 6 in the second series of cases.

In regard to the living islet donors, the operation and their courses were first described (along with a summation of the recipients courses) in a separate paper, the first ever on living pancreas donors, published as part of the proceedings of the First International Symposium on Transplantation of the Pancreas held in Lyon, France in March, 1980.[1] In the same publication the outcomes of the first three LDs of segmental pancreas grafts were described, with the courses of the first three recipients of LD pancreas recipients described in this and a companion paper on the first 12 recipients (nine deceased-donor grafts) of pancreas transplants in the new Minnesota series.[2] But the living islet-donor story comes first.

Living-Donor Islet Transplants

Both LD islet allograft recipients done at the University of Minnesota had had previous LD kidney transplants, in the first case from a different and in the second from the same sibling.[1] In the first case, we had a technical problem with the islet isolation when our mechanical tissue chopper malfunctioned during the tissue preparation and had to be repaired, resulting in prolonged ischemia. Nevertheless, the recipient became C-peptide positive after the transplant and his insulin requirements decreased, but he could not be withdrawn from insulin. He was already on azathioprine and prednisone at the time of the islet transplant because of the renal allograft placed more than three years previously and had been rejection-free, but nevertheless, since it was a different donor, he was given a course of thymoglobulin. Predictably, in this pre-antiviral drug era, at four weeks, he developed a cytomegalovirus (CMV) infection. Immunosuprression was reduced, but during the next month his C-peptide levels declined to the pre-transplant baseline, indicating the islets had failed. He subsequently (two years later) received a deceased-donor pancreas graft that functioned for five years and ultimately (24 years later) required another kidney transplant that is currently functioning, and he remains diabetic.

The second recipient of a living-donor islet allograft was severely vasculopathic and thus a better candidate for an islet than a pancreas transplant, prompting us to try again.[1] She had received a kidney allograft three years earlier from her sister and had had a severe rejection episode during the first year, so the islet allograft was done in the face of presensitization to her donor even though the crossmatch was negative with the techniques used at the time. Nevertheless, the patient became C-peptide positive and was insulin independent during the third week post-transplant, before abruptly becoming hyperglycaemic with loss of C-peptide and needing to resume exogenous insulin at her pre-transplant dose.[1,14] She died a few years later of a myocardial infarct.

Both of the LD islet allografts were considered early failures.[1] The first may have been partly for technical reasons, something we were trying to avoid so we could interpret our previous deceased-donor islet allograft results, though most likely rejection occurred after reduction in immunosuppression to allow recovery from the CMV infection.[2] Because of our experience in the second patient, we decided that related donors who had previously given a kidney should not be a donor for a pancreas or islet transplant if the prospective recipient had had a previous rejection episode of the kidney.[1]

Although the success with two of our first three islet autografts[14] had been one factor that prompted us to do the LD islet allografts, the next six islet autografts prevented insulin-dependence in only one patient.[19] We were concerned that the technical aspects of islet preparation were not satisfactorily solved, and in 1978, transplantation of immediately vascularized pancreatic deceased grafts was resumed at the University of Minnesota,[16] followed a year later by initiation of living-donor pancreas transplants,[1] as described later in this chapter.

The fact that the first two LDs of a pancreas segment for islet isolation did not have surgical complications, retained their spleens and did not develop diabetes or even glucose intolerance, encouraged us to go ahead with living-donor segmental pancreas transplants.[1] The literature on major pancreatic resections at that time indicated that most of the pancreas could be removed from a normal individual without causing diabetes,[20–22] so the outcome in our two islet donors was not surprising. However, the presumption did need to be confirmed and thus both LD islet donors and the subsequent living-pancreas donors were serially studied, a task ably carried out by our endocrinologist colleagues over the years,[23–26] allowing us to refine the criteria for living pancreas donation as we uncovered risk factors for glucose intolerance or diabetes.

Our first publication on living-related donor segmental pancreatectomy for transplantation included a table outlining the technical details of the surgery; an illustration of serial spleen scans post-donation showing an initial loss and then a regain of full function by two weeks; and the results of pre-donation and one to three years post-donation metabolic studies, including the first living islet and first living pancreas donors.[1]

However, to continue the discussion on islet transplants, as expected, technical advances over time improved the results of islet autografts so by the 1990s, with adequate yields, insulin-independence could be achieved in 70% of pancreatectomized patients if more than 300,000 islets were transplanted.[27] Although not yet achieving the efficiency of pancreas transplants[28,29] the results of islet allografts also improved over time[30] and, at least at our centre, in some cases islets from a single donor could induce insulin-independence in a recipient,[31,32] raising the possibility that living-donor islet allografts could be done again.

Indeed, a third LD islet allograft (mother to daughter, diabetic by lieu of chronic pancreatitis) has been recently reported.[33] It was carried out by Shinichi Matsumoto (a former islet research fellow at the University of Minnesota) and colleagues at the University of Kyoto on 19 January 2005, more than a quarter of a century after the second case,[1] but the one in Kyoto was successful in that the recipient was insulin-independent for at least seven months.[34,35]

In the interim, between the years of the first (1977) and most recent (2005) living-donor islet allograft (total of three cases), more than 150 living-donor segmental pancreas transplants were carried out, including 124 at the University of Minnesota. The story of the early application of living-donor segmental pancreas transplants, the circumstances prompting its application and its evolution over time, is told in the remainder of this chapter.

Living-Donor Segmental Pancreas Transplants

The first living-donor pancreas transplant was done as a segmental graft (body and tail) from a mother to her diabetic daughter at the University of Minnesota Hospital on 20 June 1979, with the duct left open.[1,2] The mother had donated a kidney to her daughter two and a half years previously, so the second donation and reception was in the pancreas after kidney (PAK) transplant category. It was the sixth pancreas transplant altogether in a new Minnesota series[2] that had begun 11 months previously, on 25 July 1978,[16] a half decade after the last case of Lillehei in his series at the same institution.[6] The LD case was reported at the March 1980 Lyon meeting as part of 12 segmental pancreas transplants that had been done in the new Minnesota series up to that time, including two more (both PAKs) from LDs.[2]

At the time of the Lyon meeting nearly all deceased-donor pancreas transplants were being done by using the segmental technique, with various methods of duct management, as can be seen by perusal of the published proceedings.[36] The duct management technique was controversial, but most centres just getting into pancreas transplantation were either using enteric drainage, as promoted by the Stockholm group,[10] or the duct-injection technique introduced by the Lyon group,[11] while at Minnesota we were leaving the pancreatic duct open to drain into the peritoneal cavity.[37] We had done segmental pancreas transplants in canines leaving the duct open as a control against duct-injection and other techniques and had found that, providing that the pancreatic enzymes remained inactive (not exposed to enterokinase) the secretions were absorbed with a remarkably low incidence of peritonitis or technical complications,[38] and thus applied the technique clinically.[12,37] The bladder drainage technique, developed by Hans Sollinger and colleagues at the University of Wisconsin,[39] as a variation of the urinary drainage technique pioneered by the Montefiore group,[9] was to come later.[40]

Although the open-duct technique was technically successful in half of our clinical cases,[2,37] and indeed our very first recipient of an open-duct deceased-donor graft done in July 1978[16] went on to enjoy insulin-independence for 17 years until she died with a functioning graft after being thrown off a horse,[17] after 13 cases, including four LD open-duct grafts,[41] it was clear that this method of exocrine drainage was tolerated better in canines than in humans and we gave it up.[42] We went on to use all duct management techniques for deceased and LD cases alike, as summarized in a 1993 article, written after > 500 total and > 75 LD pancreas transplants had been done, describing the evolution of transplantation for diabetes up to that time at the University of Minnesota.[40] Following the lead of Starzl *et al.*[43] we resumed using whole pancreaticoduodenal grafts from most deceased donors in 1985,[44] as did nearly every centre,[45] but of course LD pancreas transplants continued to be segmental.[42] (Of our 124 LD pancreas transplants through 2006,[17] exocrine secretion management was by open duct in five, duct injection in 13, enteric drainage in 57, bladder drainage in 45 and ureteral drainage in four.)

At the time of the Lyon meeting, only 105 pancreas transplants in 98 patients were known to have been done in the world,[7] and the first LD case was approximately the world's eightieth pancreas transplant since the very first.[4] At the Lyon meeting, four LD pancreas transplants were reported, the three from Minnesota[1,2] and one from Stockholm – the first LD pancreas transplant alone (PTA) – carried out by Carl Groth and associates on 18 March 1980,[46] less than two weeks before the meeting. The Stockholm recipient rejected the LD pancreas graft within a month, which was unfortunate since one of the original rationales for LD pancreas transplants was to decrease the possibility of rejection, given the high rate of early rejection in the technically successful deceased-donor pancreas transplants done to date.[7,8–12] Our initial approach of doing an LD PAK from the same donor as the kidney for a recipient with no prior rejection episodes of the kidney (and thus a confirmed non-responder to the donor) was designed to thwart the high pancreas allograft rejection rate the other groups, as well as our own,[16] were experiencing.

At the time of the Lyon meeting the first Minnesota LD pancreas transplant had been functioning nine months, and metabolic studies in the recipient showed excellent graft endocrine function. The residual pancreas of the donor also showed excellent function on metabolic testing. Our first LD pancreas transplant recipient differed from the first

Stockholm case not only by being a PAK, but a PAK from the same donor (SD) as for her renal allograft, which had not undergone any rejection episodes, a favourable situation since the recipient was demonstrably immunologically unreactive to the donor under the immunosuppressive regimen in use (in her case, Azathioprine and Prednisone). The risk of rejection was much higher for the Stockholm LD PTA case, at least as high as that of an HLA-mismatched LD kidney transplant at the time, and the risk of graft loss probably higher given that hyperglycaemia was know as a late sign of rejection in animal models, making efforts at reversal less likely to succeed.[47] Nevertheless, at Minnesota we went on to do LD PTAs within two months of the Lyon meeting,[41] while continuing to do LD PAK transplants[42] and ultimately LD (1994) SPK transplants.[17,48]

The technique of LD distal pancreastectomy was outlined at the Lyon meeting, but the first illustration of the surgical (open laparotomy) technique was published two years later,[49] after our eighth LD case (out of 35 total from July 1978 to October 1981). This publication[49] also contained data on metabolic studies in the LD pancreas donors and their recipients. Indeed, the pancreas recipient (our sixth LD case, PAK from SD, duct-injected, carried out 3 December 1980) had the longest duration of insulin-independence (23.5 years) in our series until recently eclipsed by a PTA recipient, our 24th LD case, ED, done 4 November 1982, now insulin-independent for more than 24 years.[17]

The surgical technique for LD pancreastectomy we described at the beginning of our series[1,49] remained standard[50] until 2000, when we began to do the operation laparoscopically.[51] There have been no technical failures to date (eight cases) with the laparoscopic approach, with or without concomitant donor nephrectomy.

Except for the LD PTA at Stockholm in 1980,[46] and an unpublished but registry-reported[52] single LD SPK transplant (open duct) at the University of Miami in November 1980 that failed for technical reasons, no LD pancreas transplants outside of Minnesota were published or reported to the registry until the Stockholm group did two more PTA cases in October and November 1985.[53] Neither of the second or third Stockholm LD pancreas transplants achieved long-term function but it is not clear from their publication as to the causes of loss.[53] They did publish detailed metabolic studies on the LDs that showed a decline in insulin-secretory capacity at three months with some recovery at one year, and all three Stockholm donors were insulin-independent at the time of the report.[54] After the Stockholm cases in 1985 (only the third and fourth outside of Minnesota), seven centres (one Europe, one Middle East, two USA and three Asian) either published[55,56] or reported 24 more cases as of 2006, for a total of 28 outside of Minnesota.

The most significant series of LD pancreas transplants outside of the University of Minnesota is that of Enrico Bendedetti and his colleagues at the University of Illinois in Chicago, with more than ten LD pancreas transplants to date (only seven – all SPK – reported to the registry). They have published on the results of their series[56–58] including successful transplants from identical twin donors with recurrence of disease (autoimmune destruction of beta cells) prevented by immunosuppression[57] and successful transplantation of ABO-incompatible LD pancreas-kidney transplants by antibody reduction protocols,[58] advancing the steps taken in these areas earlier at the University of Minnesota.[17,40]

It is apparent that LD pancreas transplants have been done predominantly at the University of Minnesota, 124 cases through 2006, nearly 7% of our pancreas transplants since 1978. The outcomes of and protocols for LD pancreas transplants at the University of Minnesota have been sequentially published as the series expanded,[2,16,17,22–26,37,40–42,44,48,51,59–94] now over more than a quarter of a century since the first case.[1]

The proportion of LD pancreas transplants at Minnesota has decreased with time as the results with deceased donors have got better.[17] The number of deceased donors available for solitary pancreas transplants can still meet the demand – though this scenario could change if more candidates list – but LD pancreas transplant is definitely advantageous for the sensitized candidate who finds a volunteer to whom he or she has a negative crossmatch. In addition, a LD SPK from the same donor still allows a fixed date for the transplant and a single operation to place both organs and pre-empt dialysis in the nephropathic diabetic. Although an SPK from a deceased pancreas and living-kidney donor achieves the one operation goal,[40] it does not allow a fixed date with a guarantee that a deceased-pancreas donor will be available[95,96]; an open date means the donor has to also be on call, and the probability of attaining a deceased-donor pancreas on a fixed date for a LD kidney transplant is relatively low. Thus, we offer a menu (one that has historically evolved) to the uraemic diabetic: a LD SPK with both organs from the same donor; an LD kidney on a fixed date with hope that a deceased-donor pancreas will be available and if not, subsequent to the LD kidney the recipient can be placed on the list for a deceased-donor PAK; a LD kidney done urgently when a deceased-donor pancreas is allocated to the recipient; and the waiting list for a deceased-donor SPK for both organs for those who do not have a LD for either.[17]

A few unique aspects of our LD pancreas transplant experience warrant comments or notation, including the original rationale for the procedure[1,40,42]; our observations on recurrence of autoimmune disease (selective beta-cell destruction, isletitis) in LD pancreas grafts[61,62,66,67,74,76,79,80] that were later followed by rare, but similar, observations in deceased donor grafts[97–101]; the use of parental donors for the rare paediatric recipient[40,86]; the introduction and development of laparoscopic surgery for LD segmental pancreatectomy[51,94]; the importance of metabolic studies before and after surgery in living-pancreas donors for refining the criteria to be a donor[23-26,93]; the shift in LD pancreas transplant categories from predominantly PTA and PAK to SPK cases as the results of solitary pancreas transplant improved[17,85,92] with a another shift occurring as the option of doing a SPK from a deceased pancreas and a living kidney donor[42] expanded in application[17,95,96]; the need for kidney after pancreas (KAP) transplants in some PTA recipients with LDs done for some[17,40]; the role of the registry in tracking LD pancreas transplants around the world[102]; and the ethical issues surrounding LDs, including of the pancreas,[82,103] and the need for guidelines on donor selection follow-up care.[103]

Perspectives

The rationale to use LDs for transplantation of any organ is twofold, either to get better outcomes than with deceased donors or to alleviate a shortage of deceased-donor organs, or both. Initially for pancreas transplants the main rationale was for better outcomes.

The early rationale for LD pancreas transplants was to reduce the incidence of rejection[1,40,42] and that objective was achieved[63] but more so for PAK than PTA recipients in the pre-cyclosporine (1978–84) era.[91]

In the cyclosporine era (1984–94), PTA as well as PAK immunological failures were fewer with LDs than deceased donors,[84] but after tacrolimus was introduced in 1994[85] the results of living- and deceased-donor solitary pancreas transplants were not much different.[92] Indeed we did find that technically successful graft survival rates were higher with living than deceased donors even in the early part of the new series of pancreas transplants at the University of Minnesota,[42,63] but much more so for PAK than PTA transplants, primary because the rejection rates were so much lower for same donor LD PAK than LD PTA transplants.[92] Not until the cyclosporine era were the LD PTA pancreas transplant survival rates significantly higher than those for deceased donors.[77,84] Once we began using tacrolimus the difference in outcomes between LD and deceased-donor outcomes became less.[84,92] Thus, we began doing simultaneous pancreas and kidney transplants from the same LD for recipients who wanted a fixed date and one operation for both organs,[87–94] as opposed to a fixed-date LD kidney followed by a deceased-donor PAK, or unfixed date with living-kidney donor on call for when a deceased-donor pancreas became available for a simultaneous transplant.[17,40] We have also succeeded with ABO-incompatible LD SPK transplants, the incentive being to pre-empt dialysis and correct diabetes with one operation.[17]

Initially, we had preferred sequential kidney and pancreas (PAK) transplants for the uraemic diabetic, keeping the magnitude of the operation low relative to combined placement of both organs.[2,40,42] Because we had carried out renal allografts routinely in diabetic patients during the 1970s,[18] a large recipient pool was available for both deceased and LD PAK transplants when the current Minnesota series began in 1978.[2,16,40] In 1986 we resumed SPK transplants at the University of Minnesota,[44] either with both from the same deceased donor, or with a deceased donor for the pancreas and living donor for the kidney,[40] and began doing LD SPK transplants with both organs from the same donor in March 1994.[48] The LD SPK programme rapidly expanded in the next few years.[87–94] As of 2006 we had done 38 LD SPK transplants,[17] and nine have functioned for > 10 years. During this period (1994–2006) we did only four PTAs and two PAKs from LDs, a shift in our approach compared to 1979–94 when we did 49 PTAs and 31 PAKs from LDs.[17] The shift occurred because the results of deceased-donor PTA and PAK transplants improved[92] so there was less incentive to use LDs purely for outcome, and the waiting times for solitary pancreas transplants from deceased donors remains relatively short for unsensitized candidates.

Currently at our centre LD PTA and PAK transplants are done mainly in patients who have HLA antibodies, making finding a deceased donor difficult, but who have a negative crossmatch to a suitable living-donor volunteer. In the case of LD PAK transplants, they can be from the same or different donor. The SD does give an immunological advantage, but we have recipients in both categories with long-term function.

The recurrence of disease in pancreas transplants was a surprise to us, as noted in the early citations,[61,62,66,67,74,76,78,79] but perhaps should not have been since an autoimmune etiology of type 1 diabetes was current, though still controversial. Our observations of rapid recurrence of autoimmune beta-cell destruction in non-immunosuppressed identical twin transplants was the trigger of realization,[66,67] but indeed we had already had at least two cases in immunosuppressed LD recipients,[61] and we were just uncertain of the etiology in the face of immunosuppression. It is now obvious that in some recipients of pancreas grafts, the autoimmune response to beta cells is greater than to the histocompatibilty antigens, given that recurrence of disease occurs in a percentage of recipients of deceased[97–101] as well as LD pancreas transplants.

Pancreas transplantation in children is rare, but diabetic children may develop renal disease independent of diabetes and thus be candidates for an SPK or PAK, and with severe lability for a PTA. We have carried out transplantations in children in the SPK and PTA categories, with one each from LD,[42,86] both with parenteral donors. Although the LD PTA graft from the father functioned only five years, the recipient (type 1 diabetes) thereafter was no longer labile, so the transplant served its purpose to get him through adolescence and beyond. The pancreas graft in the LD SPK case (diabetes and renal failure secondary to haemolytic uraemic syndrome is still functioning at > 11 years, though a kidney re-transplant was required at nine years. We remain open to doing more paediatric pancreas transplants with LDs.

In regard to LDs of pancreas segments, our first concern is having the least surgical complications possible and our second and equal is selecting volunteers who have sufficient beta-cell mass to stay non-diabetic post-donation. The technical complications rate has been low and the laparoscopic approach allows rapid recovery.[94] However, the metabolic effect of hemi-pancreatectomy is less predictable[23–26] than we originally thought,[1] and 3–5% of donors may eventually become diabetic even with the current criteria outlined in. We continue to work with our endocrinologists to find the screening tests that will lower the risk. Currently we use the criteria as outlined in the Vancouver forum on living donors.[103]

The future of LD pancreas or islet transplants remains uncertain. The short waiting time for deceased-donor solitary pancreas transplants currently limits the incentive of LDs, though that may change since there is little reason for PAK candidates not to list, and PTA transplants are probably also under-utilized. A deceased-donor shortage could trigger a resurgence of LD solitary pancreas transplants. There are alternatives to LD SPK transplants with the use of LD kidney and deceased-donor pancreas, simultaneously or sequentially, but again, a shortage of deceased donors could increase the incentive for same-donor LD SPK transplants.

The history of pancreas transplantation is in its fourth decade, with living pancreas donors used nearly two-thirds of that time.[104] We think the application will continue.

References

1. Sutherland DERS, Goetz FC, Najarian JS. Living related donor segmental pancreatectomy for transplantation. *Transplant. Proc.* 1980;12(2):19–25.
2. Sutherland DER, Goetz FC, Najarian JS. Report of 12 clinical cases of segmental pancreas transplantation at the University of Minnesota. *Transplant. Proc.* 1980;12(4,2):33–9.
3. Deterling R. Comment on living-donor intestinal transplantations. In Alican F, Hardy JD, Cayirli M, *et al.* Intestinal transplantation: laboratory experience and report of a clinical case. *Am. J. Surg.* 1971;121:150–9.
4. Kelly WD, Lillehei RC, Markel FK, Idezuki Y, Goetz FC. Allotransplantation of the pancreas and duodenum along with the kidney in diabetic nephropathy. *Surgery* 1967;61:827–35.
5. Lillehei RC, Simmons RL, Najarian JS, Weil R, Uchida H, Ruiz JO, Kjellstrand CM, Goetz FC. Pancreatico-duodenal allotransplantation: experimental and clinical experience. *Ann. Surg.* 1970;172:405–36.

6. Lillehei RC, Ruiz JO, Aquino C, Goetz FC. Transplantation of the pancreas. *Acta Endocrinol.* 1976;83(205):303–20.
7. Sutherland DER. International human pancreas and islet transplant registry. *Transplant. Proc.* 1980;12(4,2):229–36.
8. Connolly JE, Martin RC, Steinberg J, *et al.* Clinical experience with pancreaticoduodenal transplantation. *Arch. Surg.* 1973;106:489–93.
9. Gliedman ML, Gold M, Whittaker J, Rifkin H, Sobreman R, Freed S, Tellis V, Veith FJ. Clinical segmental pancreatic transplantation with ureter-pancreatic duct anastomosis for exocrine drainage. *Surgery* 1973;74:171–80.
10. Groth CG, Lundgren G, Arner P, Collste H, Hardsted C, Lewander R Ostman J. Rejection of isolated pancreatic allografts in patients with diabetes. *Surg. Gynecol. Obstet.* 1976;143:933–7.
11. Dubernard JM, Traeger J, Neyra P, Touraine JL, Traudiant D, Blanc-Brunat N. A new method of preparation of segmental pancreatic grafts for transplantation: trials in dogs and in man. *Surgery* 1978;84:633–40.
12. Najarian JS, Sutherland DER, Matas AJ, Steffes MW, Simmons RL, Goetz FC. Human islet transplantation: a preliminary experience. *Transplant. Proc.* 1977;9:233–6.
13. Sutherland DERS, Matas AJ, Najarian JS. Pancreatic islet cell transplantation. *Surg. Clin. N. Am.* 1978;58:365–82.
14. Sutherland DER, Matas AJ, Goetz FC, Najarian JS. Transplantation of dispersed pancreatic islet tissue in humans: autografts and allografts. *Diabetes* 1980;29:31–4.
15. Hering BJ, Kandaswamy R, Ansite JD, *et al.* Single-donor, marginal-dose islet transplantation in patients with type 1 diabetes. *JAMA* 2005;293:830–5.
16. Sutherland DER, Goetz FC, Najarian JS. Intraperitoneal transplantation of immediately vascularized segmental pancreatic grafts without duct ligation: a clinical trial. *Transplantation* 1979;28:485–91.
17. Sutherland DER, Gruessner RW, Dunn DL, Matas AJ, Humar A, Kandaswamy R, Mauer SM, Kennedy WR, Goetz FC, Robertson RP, Gruessner AC, Najarian JS. Pancreas transplantation at the University of Minnesota: 1966–2005. In *Pancreatic Transplantation.* Eds: RJ Corry, R Shapiro. New York: Informa Healthcare. 2007, pp 279–332.
18. Najarian JS, Sutherland DER, Simmons RL, Howard RJ, Kjellstrand CM, Ramsay RC, Goetz FC, Fryd DS, Sommer BG. Ten-year experience with

renal transplantation in juvenile-onset diabetics. *Ann. Surg.* 1979;190: 487–500.

19. Najarian JS, Sutherland DER, Baumgartner D, Burke B, Rynasiewicz JJ, Matas AJ, Goetz FC. Total or near total pancreatectomy and islet autotransplantation for treatment of chronic pancreatitis. *Ann. Surg.* 1980; 192:526–42.
20. Yellin AE, Vecchione TR, Donovan AJ. Distal pancreatectomy for pancreatic trauma. *Am. J. Surg.* 1972;124:135–41.
21. Stephanini P, Carboni M, Patrassi N, Basoli A. Beta-islet tumors of the pancreas: results of a study on 1,077 cases. *Surgery* 1974;75:597–609.
22. Griffin W. In *Metabolic Surgery*. Eds: H Buchwald, RC Varco. New York: Grune & Stratton. 1978, p 111.
23. Kendall DM, Sutherland DER, Goetz FC, Najarian JS. Metabolic effect of hemipancreatectomy in living related pancreas transplant donors: preoperative prediction of postoperative oral glucose tolerance. *Diabetes* 1989;38(1):101–3.
24. Kendall DM, Sutherland DER, Najarian JS, Goetz FC, Robertson, RP. Effects of hemipancreatectomy on insulin secretion and glucose tolerance in healthy humans. *New Engl. J. Med.* 1990;322:898–903.
25. Seaquist ER, Robertson RP. Effects of hemipancreatectomy on pancreatic alpha- and beta-cell function in healthy human donors. *J. Clin. Invest.* 1992;89:1761–6.
26. Robertson RP, Sutherland DE, Seaquist ER, Lanz KJ. Glucagon, catecholamine, and symptom responses to hypoglycemia in living donors of pancreas segments. *Diabetes* 2003;52:1689–94.
27. Wahoff DC, Papalois B, Najarian JS, *et al.* Autologous islet transplantation to prevent diabetes after pancreatic resections. *Ann. Surg.* 1995;222(4): 562–79.
28. Frank AM, Barker CF, Markmann JF. Comparison of whole pancreas and isolated islet transplantation for type 1 diabetes mellitus. Chapter 7. *Adv. Surg.* 2005;39:137–62.
29. Sutherland, DER. Beta-cell replacement by transplantation in diabetes mellitus: which patients at what risk, which way (when pancreas, when islets), and how to allocate deceased-donor pancreases. *Curr. Opin. Organ Transplant.* 2005;10:147–9.

30. Merani S, Shapiro AMJ. Current status of pancreatic islet transplantation. *Clin. Sci.* 2006;110:611–25.
31. Gores PF, Najarian JS, Stephania E, Lloveras JJ, Kelley SL, Sutherland DER. Insulin-independence in type 1 diabetes after transplantation of unpurified islets from a single donor using 15-deoxyspergualin. *Lancet* 1993;34:19–21.
32. Hering BJ, Kandaswamy Harmon JV, *et al.* Transplantation of cultured islets from two-layer preserved pancreases in type 1 diabetes with anti-CD3 antibody. *Am. J. Transplant.* 2004;4:390–401.
33. Matsumoto S, Okitsu T, Iwanaga Y, Noguchi H, Nagata H, Yonekawa Y, Yamada Y, Fukuda K, Tsukiyama K, Suzuki H, *et al.* Insulin-independence after living-donor distal pancreatectomy and islet allotransplantation. *Lancet* 2005;365(9471):1642–4.
34. Matsumoto S, Okitsu T, Iwanaga Y, Noguchi H, Nagata H, Yonekawa Y, Yamada Y, Nakai Y, Ueda M, Ishii A, *et al.* Insulin-independence of unstable diabetic patient after single living-donor islet transplantation. *Transplant. Proc.* 2005;37(8):3427–9.
35. Matsumoto S, Okitsu T, Iwanaga Y, Noguchi H, Yonekawa Y, Liu X, Nakai Y, Ueda M, Nagata H. Follow-up study of the first successful living-donor islet transplantation. *Am. J. Transplant. Suppl.* 2006; World Transplant Congress abstract No. 808, p. 339.
36. Dubernard JM, Traeger J (eds), *Transplantation of the Pancreas*. New York: Grune and Stratton. 1981. Hardcover edition of the December 1980 issue (Vol. XII, No. 4, Suppl. 2) of the *J. Transplant. Proc.*
37. Sutherland DER, Baumgartner D, Najarian JS. Free intraperitoneal drainage of segmental pancreas grafts: clinical and experimental observations on technical aspects. *Transplant. Proc.* 1980;12(4,2):26–32.
38. Baumgartner D, Sutherland DER, Najarian JS. Studies on segmental pancreas autotransplants in dogs. Technique and preservation. *Transplant. Proc.* 1980;12(4,2):163–171.
39. Sollinger HW, Cook K, Kamps D. Clinical and experimental experience with pancreaticocystostomy for exocrine drainage in pancreas transplantation. *Transplant. Proc.* 1984;16:749–51.
40. Sutherland DER, Gores PF, Farney C, Wahoff DC, Matas AJ, Dunn DL, Gruessner RWG, Najarian JS. Evolution of kidney, pancreas and islet

transplantation for patients with diabetes at the University of Minnesota. *Am. J. Surg.* 1993;166:456–91.
41. Sutherland DER, Goetz FC, Najarian JS. Review of the world's experience with pancreas and islet transplantation and results of intraperitoneal segmental pancreas transplantation from related and cadaver donors at Minnesota. *Transplant. Proc.* 1981;13:291–7.
42. Sutherland DER, Goetz FC, Rynasiewicz JJ, Baumgartner D, White DC, Elick BA, Najarian JS. Segmental pancreas transplantation from living related and cadaver donors: a clinical experience. *Surgery* 1981;90:159–69.
43. Starzl TE, Iwatsuki S, Shaw BW, Jr, Greene DA, Van Thiel DH, Nalesnik MA, Nusbacher J, Diliz-Pere H, Hakala TR. Pancreaticoduodenal transplantation in humans. *Surg. Gynecol. Obstet.* 1984:159:265–72.
44. Sutherland DER, Dunn DL, Goetz FC, Kennedy WR, Ramsay RC, Steffes MW, Mauer SM, Gruessner RW, Moudry-Munns KC, Morel P, Viste AB, Robertson RP, Najarian JS. A ten-year experience with 290 pancreas transplants at a single institution. *Ann. Surg.* 1989;210:274–85.
45. Sutherland DER, Sutherland DER, Chow SY, Moudry-Munns, KC. International Pancreas Transplant Registry report 1988. *Clin. Transplant.* 1989;3:129–49.
46. Groth CG, Lundgren G, Gunnarsson R, Hardstedt C, Ostman J. Experience with nine segmental pancreatic transplantations in preuremic diabetic patients in Stockholm. *Transplant. Proc.* 1980;12(2):68–71.
47. Sutherland DER. Pancreas and islet transplantation. 1. Experimental studies. *Diabetelogia* 1981;20:161–85.
48. Gruessner RWG, Sutherland DER. Simultaneous kidney and segmental pancreas transplants from living related donors – the first two successful cases. *Transplantation* 1996;61:1265–8.
49. Sutherland DER, Goetz FC, Elick BA, Najarian JS. Pancreas and islet transplantation in diabetic patients with long-term follow-up in selected cases. In *Proceedings of the Diabetic Renal-Retinal Syndrome, Prevention and Management.* Eds: EA Friedman, FA L'Esperance. New York: Grune & Stratton. 1982, pp 463–94.
50. Sutherland DER, Ascher NL. Distal pancreas donation from a living relative. In *Manual of Vascular Access, Organ Donation, and Transplantation.* Eds: RL Simmons, ME Finch, NL Ascher, JS Najarian. New York: Springer-Verlag. 1984, pp 153–64.

51. Gruessner RW, Kandaswamy R, Denny R. Laparoscopic simultaneous nephrectomy and distal pancreatectomy from a live donor. *J. Am. Coll. Surg.* 2001;193:333–7.
52. Sutherland DER. Pancreas and islet transplantation. II. Clinical trials. *Diabetologia* 1981;20:435–50.
53. Groth CG, Tyden G. Segmental pancreatic transplantation with enteric drainage. In *Pancreatic Transplantation.* Ed: CG Groth. London: Grune & Stratton. 1988, pp 99–112.
54. Bolinder J, Gunnarson R, Tyden G, Brattstrom C, Groth CG. Metabolic effects of living related pancreatic graft donation. *Transplant. Proc.* 1988;20(3):4475–8.
55. Abouna GM. Current status of pancreas transplantation for the treatment of diabetes mellitus. *J. Kuwait Med. Assoc.* 1997(Dec);29(4):394–5.
56. Zielinski A, Nazarewski S, Bogetti D, Sileri P, Testa G, Sankary H, Benedetti E. Simultaneous pancreas-kidney transplant from living related donor: a single-centre experience. *Transplantation* 2003;76: 547–52.
57. Benedetti E, Dunn T, Massad MG, Raofi V, Bartholomew A, Gruessner RW, Brecklin C. Successful living related simultaneous pancreas-kidney transplant between identical twins. *Transplantation* 1999;67:915–18.
58. Sammartino C, Pham T, Panaro F, Bogetti D, Jarzembowski T, Sankary H, Morelli N, Testa G, Benedetti E. Successful simultaneous pancreas-kidney transplantation from living related donor against positive crossmatch. *Am. J. Transplant.* 2004;4:140–3.
59. Sutherland DER, Najarian JS, Greenberg BZ, Senske BJ, Anderson GE, Francis RS, Goetz FC. Hormonal and metabolic effects of a pancreatic endocrine graft: vascularized segmental transplantation in insulin-dependent diabetic patients. *Ann. Intern. Med.* 1981;95:537–41.
60. Rynasiewicz JJ, Sutherland DER, Ferguson RM, *et al.* Cyclospoin A for immunosuppression: observations in rat heart, pancreas and islet allograft models and in human renal and pancreas transplantation. *Diabetes* 1982;31(4):92–108.
61. Sutherland DER, Goetz FC, Elick BA, Najarian JS. Experience with 49 segmental pancreas transplants in 45 diabetic patients. *Transplantation* 1982;34:330–8.

62. Sutherland DER, Sibley, RK, Chinn P, Xu X-Z, Michael A, Srikanta, Taub F, Najarian JS, Goetz FC. Identical twin pancreas transplants: reversal and recurrence of pathogenisis in type 1 diabetes. *Clin. Res.* 1984; 32(2):561A.
63. Sutherland DER, Goetz FC, Najarian JS. Pancreas transplants from living related donors. *Transplantation* 1984;38:625–33.
64. Sutherland DER, Goetz FC, Najarian JS. One hundred pancreas transplants at a single institution. *Ann. Surg.* 1984;200:414–40.
65. Sutherland DER, Goetz FC, Najarian JS. Recent experience with 89 pancreas transplants at a single institution. *Diabetologia* 1984;27:149–53.
66. Sutherland DER, Sibley RK, Xu XZ, Michael AF, Srikanta S, Taub F, Najarian JS, Goetz FC. Twin-to-twin pancreas transplantation: reversal and re-enactment of the pathogenesis of type 1 diabetes. *Trans. Assoc. Am. Physicians* 1984;97:80–7.
67. Sibley RK, Sutherland DER, Goetz FC, Michael AF. Recurrent diabetes mellitus in the pancreas iso- and allograft: a light and electron microscopic and immunohistochemical analysis of four cases. *Lab. Invest.* 1985;53: 132–44.
68. Sutherland DER, Goetz FC, Kendall DM, Najarian JS. Effect of donor source, technique, immunosuppression and presence or absence of end-stage diabetic nephropathy on outcome in pancreas transplant recipients. *Transplant. Proc.* 1985;17:325–30.
69. Sutherland DER, Goetz FC, Najarian JS. Surgery and possible complications in the living donor for the pancreas transplant, short- and long-term. In *Transplantation and Clinical Immunology XVI.* Ed: JL Touraine. Amsterdam: Elsevier Science Publishers. 1985, pp 7–15.
70. Sutherland DER, Casanova D, Sibley RK. Role of pancreas graft biopsies in the diagnosis and treatment of rejection after pancreas transplantation. *Transplant. Proc.* 1987;19:2329–31.
71. Prieto M, Sutherland DER, Fernandez-Cruz L, Heil JE, Najarian JS. Experimental and clinical experience with urine amylase monitoring for early diagnosis of rejection in pancreas transplantation. *Transplantation* 1987;43:71–9.
72. Prieto M, Sutherland DER, Goetz FC, Rosenberg ME, Najarian JS. Pancreas transplant results according to the technique of duct management: bladder versus enteric drainage. *Surgery* 1987;102:680–91.

73. Prieto M, Sutherland DER, Fernandez-Cruz L, Heil JE, Najarian JS. Experimental and clinical experience with urine amylase monitoring for early diagnosis of rejection in pancreas transplantation. *Transplantation* 1987;43:71–9.
74. Sibley RK, Sutherland DER. Pancreas transplantation: an immunohistologic and histopathologic examination of 100 grafts. *Am. J. Pathol.* 1987; 128:151–70.
75. Sutherland DER, Goetz FC, Najarian JS. Experience with single pancreas transplantation compared with pancreas transplantation after a kidney transplantation; and with transplantation with pancreas grafts from living related compared with cadaveric donors. In *Pancreatic Transplantation.* Ed: CG Groth. London: Grune & Stratton. 1988, pp 175–89.
76. Sibley R, Sutherland DER. Recurrence of diabetes mellitus in the pancreas graft. In *Pancreatic Transplantation.* Ed: CG Groth. London: Grune & Stratton. 1988, pp 339–55.
77. Sutherland DER, Kendall DM, Moudry KC, Navarro X, Kennedy WR, Ramsay RC, Steffes MW, Mauer SM, Goetz FC, Dunn DL, Najarian JS. Pancreas transplantation in non-uremic, type 1 diabetic recipients. *Surgery* 1988;104:453–64.
78. Sutherland DER, Sibley RK. Recurrence of disease in pancreas transplants. Chapter 2. In *Transplantation of the Endocrine Pancreas in Diabetes Mellitus.* Eds: R Van Schilfgaarde, MA Hardy. Amsterdam: Elsevier Science Publishers. 1988, pp 60–6.
79. Sutherland DER, Goetz FC, Sibley RK. Recurrence of disease in pancreas transplants. *Diabetes* 1989;38(1):85–7.
80. Nakhleh RE, Gruessner RWG, Swanson PE, *et al.* Pancreas transplant pathology. A morphologic, immunohistochemical and electron microscopic comparison of allogeneic grafts with rejection syngeneic grafts, and chronic pancreatitis. *Am. J. Surg. Pathol.* 1991;15:246–56.
81. Sutherland DER, Goetz FC, Kendall DM, Robertson RP, Gillingham KJ, Moudry-Munns KC, Najarian JS. Experience with pancreas transplants from living related donors. In *Organ Transplantation 1990.* Eds: GM Abouna, MSA Kumar, AG White. Dordrecht, The Netherlands: Kluwer Academic Publishers. 1991, pp 383–8.
82. Sutherland DER, Goetz FC, Gillingham KJ, Moudry-Munns KC, Najarian JS. Medical risks and benefit of pancreas transplants from living related

donors. In *Organ Replacement Therapy: Ethics, Justice and Commerce.* Eds: W Land, JB Dossetor. Berlin, Heidelberg: Springer-Verlag. 1991, pp 93–101.

83. Santamaria P, Nakhleh RE, Sutherland DER, Barbosa JJ. Characterization of T-lymphocytes infiltrating human pancreas allograft affected by isletitis and recurrent diabetes. *Diabetes* 1992;41:53–61.
84. Sutherland DER, Gruessner RWG, Moudry-Munns KC, Gruessner A, Najarian JS. Pancreas transplants from living related donors. *Transplant. Proc.* 1994;26(2):443–5.
85. Gruessner RWG, Sutherland DER, Najarian JS, Dunn DL, Gruessner A. Solitary pancreas transplantation for non-uremic patients with labile insulin-dependent diabetes mellitus. *Transplantation* 1997;64:1572–7.
86. Bendel-Stenzel MR, Kashtan CE, Sutherland DER, Chavers BM. Simultaneous pancreas-kidney transplant in two children with hemolytic-uremic symptom. *Pediatr. Nephrol.* 1997;11:485–7.
87. Gruessner RWG, Kendall DM, Drangstveit MB, Gruessner A, Sutherland DER. Simultaneous pancreas-kidney transplantation from live donors. *Ann. Surg.* 1997;226:471–82.
88. Humar A, Gruessner RWG, Sutherland DER. Living related donor pancreas and pancreas-kidney transplantation. *Br. Med. Bull.* 1997;53: 879–91.
89. Gruessner RWG, Leone JP, Sutherland DER. Combined kidney and pancreas transplants from living donors. *Transplant. Proc.* 1998;30:282.
90. Sutherland DER, Najarian JS, Gruessner RWG. Living- versus cadaver-donor pancreas transplants. *Transplant. Proc.* 1998;30:2264–6.
91. Kandaswamy R, Stillman AE, Granger DK, Sutherland DER, Gruessner RWG. MRI is superior to angiography for evaluation of living related simultaneous pancreas and kidney donors. *Transplant. Proc.* 1999;31: 604–5.
92. Sutherland DE, Gruessner RW, Dunn DL, Mata AJ, Humar A, Kandaswamy R, Mauer SM, Kennedy WR, Goetz FC, Robertson RP, Gruessner AC, Najarian JS. Lessons learned from more than 1,000 pancreas transplants at a single institution. *Ann. Surg.* 2001;233:463–501.
93. Gruessner RW, Sutherland DE, Drangstveit MB, Bland BJ, Gruessner AC. Pancreas transplants from living donors: short- and long-term outcome. *Transplant. Proc.* 2001;33:819–20.

94. Tan M, Kandaswamy R, Sutherland DE, Gruessner RW. Laparoscopic donor distal pancreatectomy for living-donor pancreas and pancreas-kidney transplantation. *Am. J. Transplant.* 2005;5:1966–70.
95. Farney AC, Cho E, Schweitzer EJ, Dunkin B, Philosophe B, Colonna J, Jacobs S, Jarrell B, Flowers JL, Bartlett ST. Simultaneous cadaver pancreas living-donor kidney transplantation: a new approach for the type 1 diabetic uremic patient. *Ann. Surg.* 2000;232:696.
96. Boggi U, Vistoli F, Del Chiaro M, Signori S, Coletti L, Morelli L, Pietrabissa A, Moretto C, Barsotti M, Marchetti P, Rizzo G, Mosca F. Simultaneous cadaver pancreas living-donor kidney transplantation. *Transplant. Proc.* 2004;36:577.
97. Tyden G, Reinholt FP, Sundkvist G, Bolinder J. Recurrence of autoimmune diabetes mellitus in recipients of cadaveric pancreatic grafts (see comments) (published erratum appears in *N. Engl. J. Med.* 1996 Dec 5;335(23): 1778). *N. Engl. J. Med.* 1996;335:860–3.
98. Burke GW, Ciancio G, Miller J, Allende G, Pugliese A. Hyperglycemia occurring 5–8 years after simultaneous pancreas-kidney (SPK) transplantation associated with the prior development of islet-cell antibodies. *Am. J. Transplant.* 2003;380(3):A889.
99. Pugliese A, Allende G, Laughlin R, Dogra R, Ciancio G, Miller J, Nepom GT, Burke GW. Reurrence of autoantibodies and autorreactive T-cells in patients with type 1 diabetes following pancreas transplantation. *Diabetes* 2004;53(2):A69.
100. Sisino G, Dogra R, Allende G, Dominguez-Bendala J, Ricordi C, Burk GW, Pugliese A. Evidence for ductal cell to ß-cell trans-differentiation and proliferation in the transplanted pancreas of patients with type 1 diabetes and recurrence of islet autoimmunity. *Diabetes* 2006;55(1):A32.
101. Reijonen H, Geubtner K, Allende G, Kwok W, Nepom G, Burke G, Pugliese A. Identification of islet-autoantigen specific CD4+ T-cells in the pancreatic lymph nodes and pancreas of a pancreas-kidney transplant patient with recurrence of autoimmunity. *Diabetes* 2006;55(1):A88.
102. Gruessner AC, Sutherland DE. Pancreas transplant outcomes for United States (US) and non-US cases as reported to the United Network for Organ Sharing (UNOS) and the International Pancreas Transplant Registry (IPTR) as of June 2004. *Clin. Transplant.* 2005;19:433–55.

103. Pruett TL, Tibell A, Albdulkareem A, Bhandari M, Cronin DC, Dew MA, Dob-Kuri A, Gutmann T, Matas A, McMurdo L, Rahmel A, Rizvi SAH, Wright L, Delmonico FL. The ethics statement of the Vancouver forum on live lung, liver, pancreas and intestine donor. *Transplantation* 2006;81: 1386.
104. Sutherland DER, Gruessner RWG. History of pancreas transplantation. In *Transplantation of the Pancreas.* Eds: RWG Gruessner, DER Sutherland. New York: Springer-Verlag. 2004, pp 39–68.

Chapter 5

Living Donor Small Bowel Transplantation World Experience and Register

Enrico Benedetti, Giuliano Testa, Fabrizio Panaro and Nicola Morelli

Introduction

In the last decade isolated intestinal transplantation (IT) has become a valuable surgical option to treat selected patients affected by irreversible intestinal failure (IF).[1–6] Total parenteral nutrition (TPN) represents the first therapeutic line in the management of this disease. Patients who develop life-threatening complications such as cholestatic liver disease, lack of central line access and recurrent infections should be considered for IT.

Currently cadaveric small bowel transplantation is associated with satisfactory outcomes. However, the procedure continues to be plagued by high incidence of infections, rejection and post-transplant lymphoproliferative disease (PTLD).

Theoretically, the relatively small number of candidates for IT could be easily treated using cadaveric bowel donors. In reality, the waiting time is relatively long and associated with high mortality especially for paediatric patients (see Table 1).[7,8]

The reason for this discrepancy between the potentially available donors (12,227 in the US in 2001) versus the number of bowel transplants performed (111 in 2001) is multifactorial.[7]

Table 1: Mean time and mortality on the waiting list, US (2001).[8]

Age groups (Years)	Waiting time (Days)	Mortality in waiting list (%)
0–5	177	36.7
5–18	438	11.6
Over 18	104	12.3

While HLA matching is not an obstacle as it is for other organs, the majority of centres are willing to consider only young, haemodynamically stable, size-matched donors, which are preferably CMV negative.

Living related small bowel transplantation (LR-SBTx) can minimize waiting time and prevents progression of cholestatic liver disease and mortality, which are not uncommon on the waiting list.

The Intestinal Transplant Registry (ITR) data suggest that patient and graft survival after LR-SBTx is comparable to those obtained with cadaveric donors. However LR-SBTx can theoretically offer advantages compared to whole small bowel transplantation from cadaveric donors (Table 2).

Clearly the main advantages are the marked reduction of waiting time, and the reduced mortality on the waiting list. Reduced cold ischemia time, better tissue matching and better donor's graft preparation may also represent important additional advantages.

In addition, recipient medical conditions can be optimized and since the donor is a healthy individual, haemodynamic instability and consequent pre-procurement graft hypoperfusion in the donor are obviated. All these benefits may allow an easier management of LR-SBTx recipients while providing an adequate segment of bowel to support physiologic alimentation. The main disadvantage remains the risks for the donor, which include both early and long-term surgical complications of bowel resections as well as potential long-term impairment of intestinal absorption. Other potentially detrimental factors include the functional limitation related to the necessary use of a shorter graft and the increased risk of vascular thrombosis related to the smaller vascular pedicle in the recipient.[9]

Table 2: Comparison between living-related small bowel transplantation and cadaveric intestinal transplant.

LR-SBTx	IT
Advantages	*Disadvantages*
• Elimination of waiting time	• Long waiting time
• Optimal HLA matching	• Inferior HLA matching
• Short cold ischemia time	• Long cold ischemia time
• Optimal bowel graft decontamination	• Inferior bowel graft decontamination
• Elective surgery	• Emergency surgery
Disadvantages	*Advantages*
• Risk for donor	• Donor risk n/a
• Shorter bowel graft	• Whole bowel graft
• Small vascular pedicle	• Good vascular patches

LR-SBtx represents a field in continuous evolution and its relative value in the treatment of intestinal failure has yet to be fully determined.

Indications

The indications for the LR-SBTx are the same as for isolated cadaveric bowel transplantation.

Short Bowel Syndrome (SBS) progressing to irreversible intestinal failure with inadequate absorption of fluid and nutrients represents the baseline indication for small bowel transplantation. After the introduction of total parenteral nutrition (TPN) by Dudrick in 1968, the survival of patients with SBS has remarkably improved.[10]

Nevertheless, long-term use of TPN typically leads to one or more of several complications such as recurrent episodes of central line infections, extended central vein thrombosis, lack of central venous access sites, sepsis and rapidly progressive cholestatic liver disease.

Intestinal transplantation emerged as a treatment for IF after the advent of tacrolimus in 1990. Despite its progress and recent advances, IT is a therapeutic option only for patients with IF whose condition continues to decline despite TPN therapy. IT is not yet an alternative for patients who are doing well on TPN. Three-year patient survival after isolated IT is approximately 70% which is appreciably better than in earlier eras, but is still not comparable with the three-year survival rate of at-home, stable, TPN-treated patients (90%). Patients failing TPN therapy, however, have a very poor prognosis (< 20% one-year survival).[11,12]

In this select group of patients with TPN-dependence and life-threatening complications from TPN, IT does offer a clear survival advantage. Patients who are failing while on TPN should be referred early for evaluation for IT to increase the likelihood of a successful outcome. Timely referral also decreases the likelihood of requiring combined liver/intestine transplantation for TPN-induced liver failure. Finally, it is essential that patients with end-stage IF are cared for and managed by a multidisciplinary team at a centre that has expertise in all aspects of treatment for IF: TPN, reconstructive surgery of the bowel and IT. Especially in rapidly deteriorating paediatric candidates for bowel transplantation, a timely LR-SBTx can be life-saving.[13,14]

The main indications to small bowel transplantation in adults patients is short gut syndrome secondary to intestinal ischemia or trauma due to superior mesenteric artery thrombosis or bleeding, Crohn's disease and intra-abdominal desmoid tumour.

In children the main indications for small bowel transplant are congenital diseases such as gastroschisis, volvulus and intestinal atresia (Table 3).

Table 3: Indications for small bowel transplantation.[15]

Children		Adults	
Gastroschisis	21%	Intestinal ischemia	22%
Volvulus	18%	Crohn's disease	13%
Necrotizing enterocolitis	12%	Intestinal trauma	12%
Pseudoobstruction	9%	Intra-abdominal desmoid tumor	10%
Intestinal atresia	7%	Short gut syndrome	7%
Hirschsprung's disease	7%	Volvulus	7%
Short gut syndrome	4%	Gardner's syndrome/ Familial polyposis	3%
Microvillus inclusion	4%		

Contraindications

The contraindications for IT have changed over time, becoming fewer as advancements have been made in the field and outcomes have improved. The only absolute contraindications include systemic malignancy, metastatic disease, AIDS, cardiopulmonary insufficiency, severe renal failure, advanced neurological dysfunction and overwhelming sepsis (Table 4). Relative contradictions are centre-specific and generally include weight (infants weighing less than 5 kg), and multiple previous abdominal surgical procedures.

Donor Evaluation

Potential living related small bowel donor selection starts with the preliminary determination of ABO blood type and Human Leukocyte Antigen (HLA).

The donor and recipient ABO blood types must be compatible. In the presence of multiple potential donors, the candidate with best HLA match is selected. Donors with a positive lymphocytotoxic crossmatch must be avoided. A careful evaluation of possible cardio-pulmonary risk factors must follow; Table 5 summarizes the critical points in the evaluation of potential donors for LR-SBTx.

The size match between the donor and recipient, critical in cadaver cases, is not important in the setting of LR-SBTx since a segment of

Table 4: Contraindications for IT.

Absolute	Relative
• Systemic malignancy	• Weight < 5 kg
• Metastatic disease	• Multiple previous surgeries
• HIV positive	
• Cardiopulmonary insufficiency	
• Severe renal failure	
• Neurological disorders	
• Sepsis	

Table 5: Living related donor evaluation for LR-SBTx.

- **Physical examination**
- **No history of intestinal surgery or infection**
- **ABO compatibility**
- **HLA determination**
- **Lymphocytotoxic crossmatch negative**
- **Gastroenterology (GI) assessment:** consultation, absorption tests (D-xylose, fecal fat), abdominal ultrasound, abdominal CT-scan, selective mesenteric superior angiography or 3-D-angio-CT-scan
- **Laboratory tests:** glucose, BUN, electrolytes, creatinine, bilirubin, alkaline phosphatase, AST, ALT, GGT, albumin, ammonia, alfa-fetoprotein, prothrombin time, partial thromboplastin time, triglycerides, vitamins A, D, E, K, B_{12}
- **Infectious disease assessment:** hepatitis screen, HIV, CMV (IgG, IgM), EBV (IgG, IgM), herpes zoster (IgA, EIA), stool culture, urine culture
- **Chest X-ray**
- **ECG**
- **Anesthesiology assessment:** consultation, anesthesia and surgical history, drug allergies
- **Psychosocial assessment:** psychiatry and psychological consultation, social worker consultation

bowel is used.[16] Many centres prefer using cytomegalovirus (CMV) negative donors because the significant association of post-transplant CMV disease and graft loss.[2,17]

In order to evaluate anatomy and patency of the donor's superior mesenteric vessels, conventional selective angiography is performed. Abdominal ultrasound and CT scan complete the study of the donor's abdomen to rule out eventual unknown associated pathologies. Recent advances in the radiologic field suggest that 3-D-angio-CT scan could be the pre-operative gold standard examination to study vascular anatomy of the donor's superior mesenteric vessels and especially of the ileocolic vessels, which will provide the blood supply to the small bowel graft. This method is becoming the standard 'one step' evaluation in our centre.

Intestinal decontamination of the graft is performed before surgery with standard mechanical procedure and during graft procurement with mycostatin and gentamicin. Antibiotic prophylaxis with intravenous cefoxitin is also administered.

Recipient Evaluation

To evaluate candidates for LR-SBTx, a detailed, multidisciplinary approach is needed to assess appropriate candidacy and to provide for the best possible outcome (Table 6). The goals of the evaluation are to define the cause and extent of IF, evaluate associated organ dysfunction and determine appropriate treatment, including surgical options or alternative

Table 6: Recipient evaluation.

Physical examination	Complete physical examination and review of systems
Medical and surgical history	Gastroenterology (GI) assessment: • gastroenterology consultation, upper- and lower-GI barium studies, gastric-emptying study (if indicated), motility testing (if indicated), absorption testing (D-xylose, fecal fat), abdominal ultrasound, stool cultures Hepatic function assessment: • laboratory tests: AST, ALT, GGTP, alkaline phosphatase bilirubin, albumin, ammonia, alpha-fetoprotein, prothrombin time, partial thromboplastin time, INR • diagnostic procedures: liver ultrasound, liver biopsy (if indicated)
Venous access assessment	• Ultrasound of great vessels for patency, number and placement of Broviac lines, number of line infections and organisms
Nutritional assessment	• Nutritional status: anthropometric measurements, weight, height, caloric intake • Nutritional support: TPN, enteral feeds, oral intake history, oral intake aversion history/behaviours • Laboratory tests: electrolytes, BUN, creatinine, triglycerides, vitamins A, D, E, K, B_{12}, thiamine
Infectious disease assessment	• Immunization history • Laboratory tests: hepatitis screen, HIV, CMV (IgM, IgG), EBV (IgM, IgG), herpes zoster (IgA, EIA), measles, mumps and rubella titers, cultures (blood, urine, quantitative stool)

(*Continued*)

Table 6: (*Continued*)

Physical examination	Complete physical examination and review of systems
Cardiac assessment	• Cardiology consultation, electrocardiogram, chest X-ray, echocardiogram
Pulmonary assessment	• Pulmonary consultation (if indicated), assessment for pulmonary complications: bronchopulmonary dysplasia, hepatopulmonary syndrome, cystic fibrosis
Anesthesiology assessment	• Anesthesiology consultation, anesthesia history, surgical history, drug allergies
Psychosocial assessment	• Psychiatry and psychological consultation, social worker consultation

medical and nutritional strategies. Transplantation is recommended only in cases of irreversible IF with established complications of TPN.[18]

Surgical Procedures

After Gruessner *et al.* described in 1997[3] a standardized technique for living related small bowel transplantation, the main technical problems associated with the procedure have been for the most part resolved.

We describe our current surgical technique, which is based on Gruessner *et al.*'s original description.

Donor operation

After midline laparotomy an intestinal graft consisting of 180–200 cm (150 cm for paediatric recipients) of distal ileum vascularized by the ileocolic artery and vein is isolated (Figs. 1 and 1A). A segment of 20 cm of distal ileum close to the ileocecal valve must be preserved to guarantee normal vitamin B_{12} absorption for the donor. The ileal graft is therefore procured starting 20 cm from the ileocecal valve going proximally and represents about one-third of the donor's entire small bowel. The right colic artery is carefully preserved to ensure good vascularization of the distal ileum. After systemic heparinization the ileocolic artery and vein

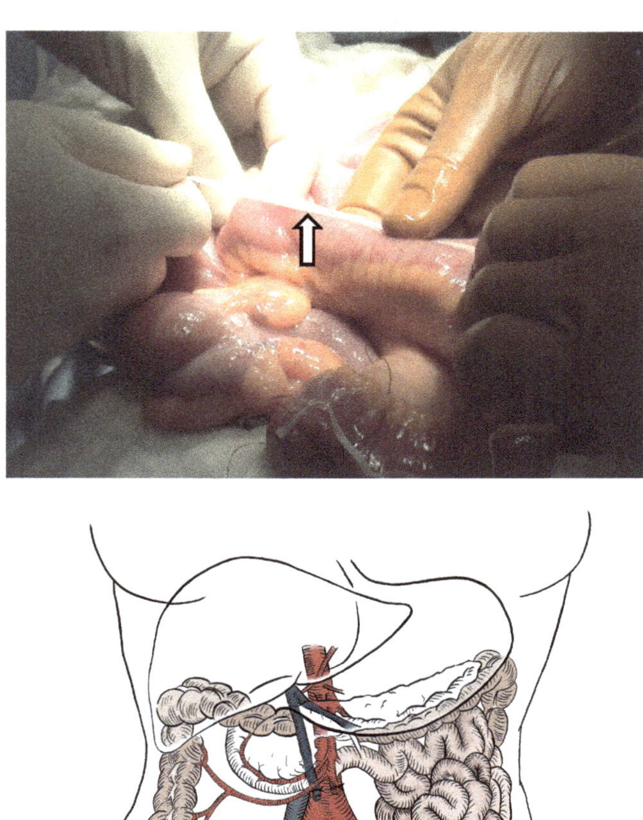

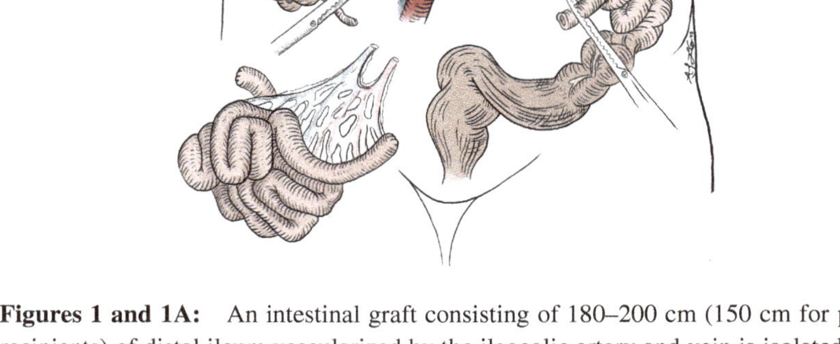

Figures 1 and 1A: An intestinal graft consisting of 180–200 cm (150 cm for pediatric recipients) of distal ileum vascularized by the ileocolic artery and vein is isolated.

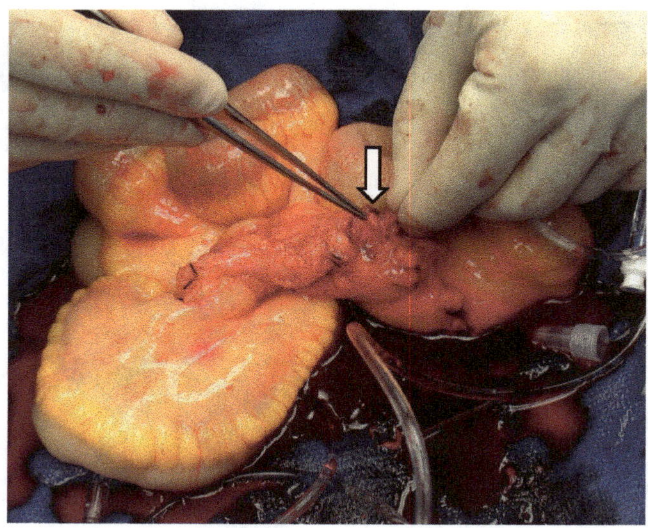

Figure 2: Graft is removed and immediately flushed with 200–250 cc of University of Wisconsin solution on the back table.

are divided just distal to the take-off of the right colic vessels. The graft is then removed and immediately flushed with 200–250 cc of University of Wisconsin solution on the back table (Fig. 2). The donor's intestinal continuity is re-established using a side-to-side intestinal stapled anastomosis.

After surgery the donor is routinely seen in the clinic 3, 6 and 12 months after surgery. At each clinic visit, a vitamin B_{12} level is obtained along with standard laboratory evaluation.

Recipient operation

After midline laparotomy and lysis of adhesions, the infrarenal aorta and cava are dissected free. If the aorta and cava dissection is difficult because of previous surgery, the right common iliac artery and vein are used as an alternative inflow for the vascular anastomosis. The ileocolic artery is anastomosed to the side of the aorta or right common iliac artery with an interrupted layer of 6-0 polypropylene sutures. The vein anastomosis is performed between the end of the ileocolic vein and the side of the vena cava

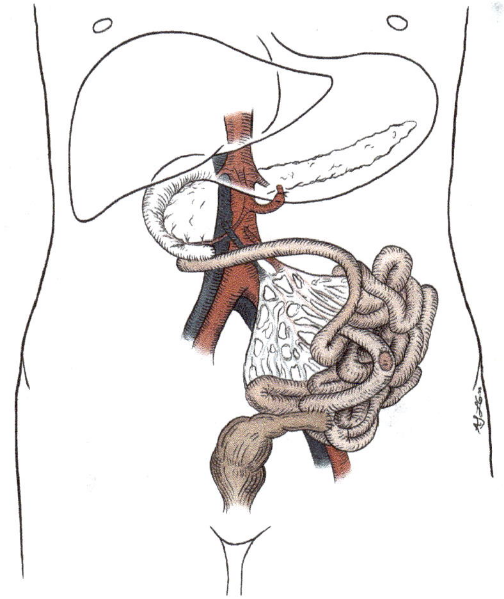

Figure 3: Vein anastomosis is performed between the end of the ileocolic vein and the side of the vena cava or right common iliac vein with running 6-0 polypropylene sutures.

or right common iliac vein with running 6-0 polypropylene sutures (Fig. 3). In our series the cold ischemic time for the graft was about ten minutes, while the warm ischemic time was 30 to 40 minutes. After reperfusion (Fig. 4), the proximal end of the intestinal graft is anastomosed side-to-side to the donor duodenum using a two-layer anastomosis with 4-0 polyglyconate for the mucosal and 4-0 polypropylene for the seromuscular layer. The distal anastomosis between the distal end of the ileal graft and the sigmoid colon is performed with a similar technique. Finally, a totally diverting loop ileostomy is performed at a distance of about 15 cm from the distal anastomosis in order to have easy access for endoscopic bowel graft biopsy and monitor the stomal output. An increase in stomal output is one of the most reliable clinical signs of graft dysfunction or rejection.

The abdominal wall closure is performed primarily in adults, while in paediatric recipients absorbable mesh is placed over the bowel and partial thickness skin graft is applied three weeks later.

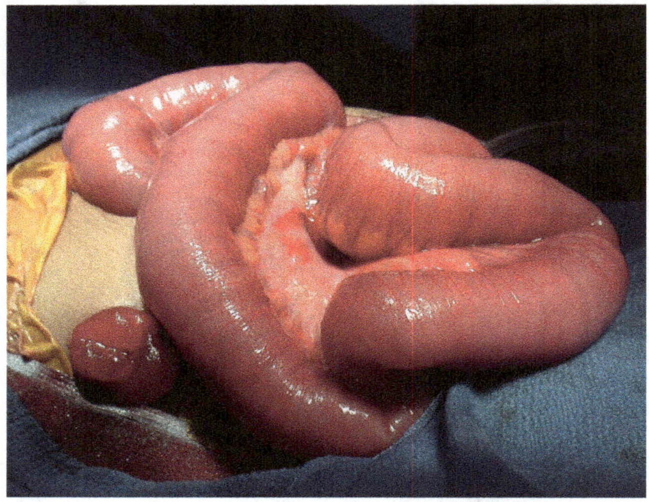

Figure 4: After reperfusion, the proximal end of the intestinal graft is anastomosed side-to-side to the donor duodenum using a two-layer anastomosis with 4-0 polyglyconate for the mucosal and 4-0 polypropylene for the seromuscular layer.

Post-Transplant Care

Management of the small bowel transplant recipient is a complex and formidable task, particularly during the first six months after transplantation. These patients are vulnerable to a wide range of complications related to rejection, infection and technical problems. The biggest challenge is achieving a balance between an adequate level of immunosuppression to prevent rejection while avoiding a heavy-handed approach that may result in infectious and neoplastic complications.[19]

Immunosuppression

Since 1990, tacrolimus (TAC) has become the primary immunosuppressant agent used in intestine transplantation, contributing to improved survival rates.[20]

TAC immunosuppression: Immunosuppression with TAC is started intraoperatively at a dose of 0.15–0.2 mg/kg/day through a continuous infusion. Oral TAC is usually begun at 3–4 times the IV dose of 0.2 mg/kg/day divided in two doses when GI motility resumes. It is often necessary to overlap dosing when changing from the IV route to the oral route, since GI absorption is unreliable during the early postoperative period. Trough levels of TAC are targeted at 20–25 ng/mL in whole blood during the early postoperative period and maintained at that range for up six months; levels are decreased to 10–15 ng/mL within 6–12 months post-transplant. Stable patients at two or more years post-transplant often have levels below 10 ng/mL.

Corticosteroids: IV methylprednisolone is given as an intraoperative bolus (10 mg/kg; maximum dose 1 g) followed by a taper over five days from 5 mg/kg/day in children or 20 mg/day in adults. Long-term immunosuppressive therapy has involved the use of TAC and steroids as well as a third agent in some patients.

Adjunctive agents: Azathioprine, mycophenolate mofetil (MMF) and sirolimus are used as adjunctive agents to treat rejection when additional immunosuppression is required or to mitigate the side effects and toxicities of TAC. Some centres have used induction therapy with OKT3, cyclophosphamide, MMF or daclizumab with varying results.[4]

Our own immunosuppressive protocol consists of a brief induction with thymoglobulin for 3–4 doses and maintenance with a combination of oral tacrolimus and prednisone. Tacrolimus doses are adjusted to achieve serum levels between 15 and 20 ng/mL during the first three months, and 5–10 ng/mL thereafter. All the recipients receive vancomycin and piperacillin peri-operatively for three days and fluconazole for one week. CMV prophylaxis is achieved using IV ganciclovir for the first week and then acyclovir for three months.

Maintaining fluid and electrolyte homeostasis

In the early postoperative period, most patients have increased interstitial accumulation of fluid in the peripheral tissues, transplanted bowel and lungs, with peak levels at 48–72 hours.[17] Careful monitoring of the renal function, electrolyte imbalances and strict measurement of intake and output are essential to appropriate management. Stomal output ranges from 40–60 cc/kg/day in children and about 1.2 litres/day in adults. Proper replacement of stomal fluid losses must continue on occasion for months.

Nutritional support

Patients receive TPN in the early postoperative period to provide nutritional support. After completion of a gastrografin swallow study to evaluate the integrity of the small bowel anastomosis and recovery of motility, TPN is weaned as enteral feedings are initiated. Patients with functional grafts can be completely weaned from TPN within 4–6 weeks postoperatively, although patients may require partial TPN during episodes of rejection and infection.[21] The Intestinal Transplant Registry (ITR) reports that 77% of recipients do not have any TPN requirement, while 14% require partial TPN support after one-year post-transplant.[15]

Assessment of graft function

Graft function is monitored following several criteria. Adequate absorption is a good indicator of satisfactory function of the transplanted intestine and is determined by serial monitoring of carbohydrate and fat absorption.[22]

However, the functional performance of the transplanted ileal graft in adults was never studied in a serial fashion. Our data suggests that, through a progressive and relatively rapid functional adaptation, a 180–200 cm ileal graft can carefully support the nutritional requirement of an active young adult.[11]

Graft function is also assessed by routine surveillance for rejection through frequent endoscopy and tissue biopsy. Stomal output is evaluated daily for volume, consistency and presence of blood and reducing substances. An increase in stomal output is one of the most reliable clinical signs of graft dysfunction or rejection.

Radiologic evaluation is done routinely through barium studies to assess the mucosal pattern of the graft motility.

Periodic endoscopic examinations with ileal graft biopsy are important in estimation of the slow graft's adaptation process (Fig. 5). The

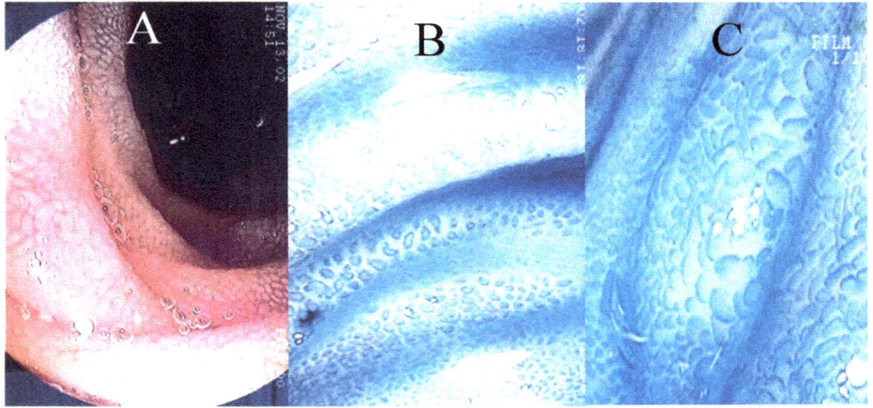

Figure 5: Periodic endoscopic examinations with ileal graft biopsy.

graft's morphologic adaptation is shown by increased villi length of at least 50% within six months (Fig. 6).[11]

As a consequence of this impressive lengthening of the villi, the absorptive surface increases by 50% by six months as well. General nutrition index, such as serum albumin levels, increase steadily after transplant and remain stable.

Postoperative Complications and Management

The worldwide experience in LR-SBTx consists only of 24 cases, 15 of which were performed in the USA. Most of the reports referred to in the literature are cases with short follow-up. No technical complications have been described.[8] In our initial experience based on eight cases of LR-SBTx, we observed only a few complications in the early postoperative course such as two early retroperitoneal bleedings and one graft necrosis three months post-transplant due to octreotide administration for acute pancreatitis.

Table 7 summarizes the most common complications after bowel transplant. The most challenging medical management task is achieving a balance between an adequate level of immunosuppression to prevent rejection, while avoiding over-immunosuppression that may result in infection.

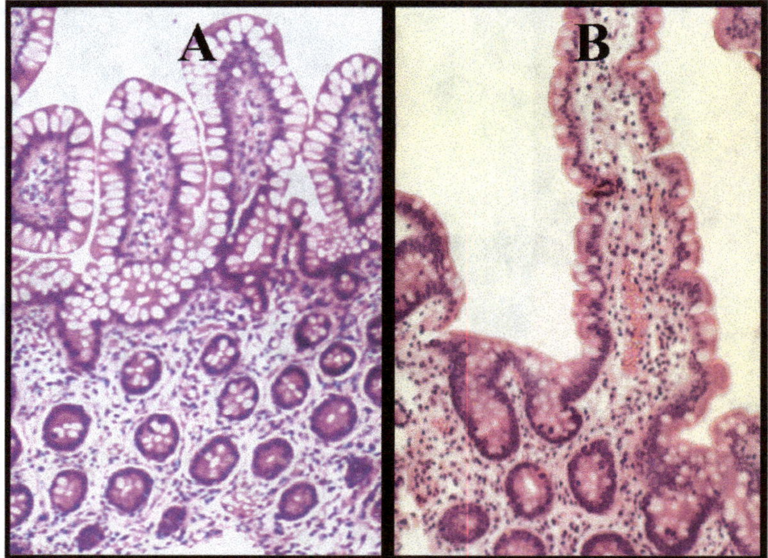

Figure 6: The graft's morphologic adaptation is shown by increased villi length of at least 50% within six months.

Table 7: Postoperative complications.

Surgical complications

- Postoperative hemorrhage
- Vascular thromboses

Gastrointestinal complications

- Bleeding
- Anastomotic leak
- Dysmotility

Rejection

- Acute
- Chronic

Infections

- Bacterial
- Fungal
- Viral

Graft-versus-host disease (GVHD)

Graft loss and re-transplantation

Rejection and treatment

Acute allograft rejection is commonly seen in cadaveric IT; the overall incidence is 78% or greater. Rejection is seen most frequently and is most severe in isolated IT (88%) as compared with combined liver/intestine grafts (66%).[12,23]

Acute rejection: Small bowel rejection ranges from a mild clinical course with minimal histologic changes, to the severe clinical picture of intractable rejection that can result in graft enterectomy or death.[12,23] Rejection is diagnosed by clinical presentation, endoscopic appearance of the bowel, and ultimately by histologic findings.

Mild-to-moderate rejection is treated by optimizing TAC level and methylprednisolone boluses. Adjunctive agents such as azathioprine, MMF, or sirolimus may also be added to the baseline regimen. In cases of refractory or severe acute rejection, anti-lymphocyte preparations (thymoglobulin, OKT3) are given.

In our experience, rejection is infrequent when a well-matched graft is used. We documented only one early rejection in our eight cases in the only graft with no HLA match. The other seven grafts with > 3 HLA match had no early rejection, although one patient had acute rejection one and half years post-transplant secondary to overt non-compliance.

Chronic rejection: Chronic rejection is a consequence of episodes of refractory acute rejection. The reported incidence of chronic rejection is 8% after cadaver bowel transplant.[18] No data in the literature is available for LR-SBTx.

Infection

Infection and sepsis are associated with high morbidity and mortality. Sepsis is the main cause of mortality after IT, usually due to high levels of immunosuppression. While the advances in immunosuppressive therapy have led to a significant reduction in the incidence of rejection, they have also set the stage for severe infectious complications of bacterial, viral, and fungal origin. Moreover, the unique nature of the intestine allows for bacterial translocation during periods of stress such as ischemia, reperfusion and rejection.[23]

Cytomegalovirus infection (CMV): One of the more common infections in IT recipients is CMV infection, which in addition to generalized CMV syndrome, can result in CMV enteritis.[18,23]

Epstein-Barr Virus (EBV) infection and PTLD: EBV and EBV-associated Post Transplant Lymphoproliferative Disorder (PTLD) are significant causes of IT-related morbidity and mortality.[19,24] The incidence of EBV-associated PTLD ranges from 5% to 23% with higher incidences documented in paediatric recipients.[12,18,23–27]

Bacteremia: Bacteremia, particularly from enteric organisms, is common after IT and is frequently noted during the ischemia-reperfusion period. The most common bacteria isolated are coagulase-negative staphylococci, enterococci, Enterobacter, Klebsiella, and Pseudomonas.[28]

Graft versus Host Disease (GVHD)

Despite the large amount of lymphoid tissue contained in intestinal grafts, the incidence of GVHD is relatively low (0–14%) and has never caused graft loss or recipient death.[4,29]

Graft loss and re-transplantation

The most common causes of graft loss are infection, rejection and technical or clinical complications.[17] Graft enterectomy should be performed if the patient has significant graft dysfunction or severe rejection that is refractory to treatment. Isolated IT patients requiring graft enterectomy will have to resume TPN should be re-listed as transplant candidates if criteria for listing are met and the patient and family desire re-transplantation.

Report from the United Network of Organ Sharing (UNOS) and the Intestinal Transplant Registry (ITR)[7–8]

The ITR was established in 1994 to review the worldwide experience for the IV International Symposium on Small Bowel Transplantation. Subsequently, a report from the ITR has been prepared every two years. Currently, 55 centers in 17 countries submit data to the ITR.

Between April 1985 and 31 May 2001, 696 transplants performed in 656 patients were reported to the ITR. Of these, 24 cases were performed using living donors. According to UNOS registry (from 1 January 1998 to 31 March 2003) in the United States to date there have been 731 total bowel transplants. Of those, 15 have been from living donors.

The overall analysis of the ITR and UNOS data allows some relevant considerations. Patient and graft survival after living related small bowel transplant is comparable to the results obtained with cadaveric donors (Tables 8 and 9).

Table 8: Graft survival – donor type.[7]

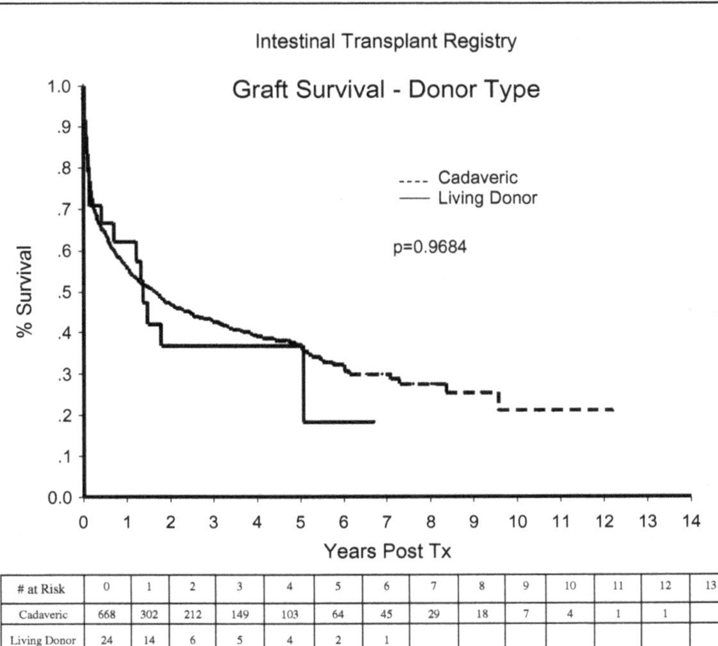

# at Risk	0	1	2	3	4	5	6	7	8	9	10	11	12	13
Cadaveric	668	302	212	149	103	64	45	29	18	7	4	1	1	
Living Donor	24	14	6	5	4	2	1							

Table 9: Patient survival – donor type.[7]

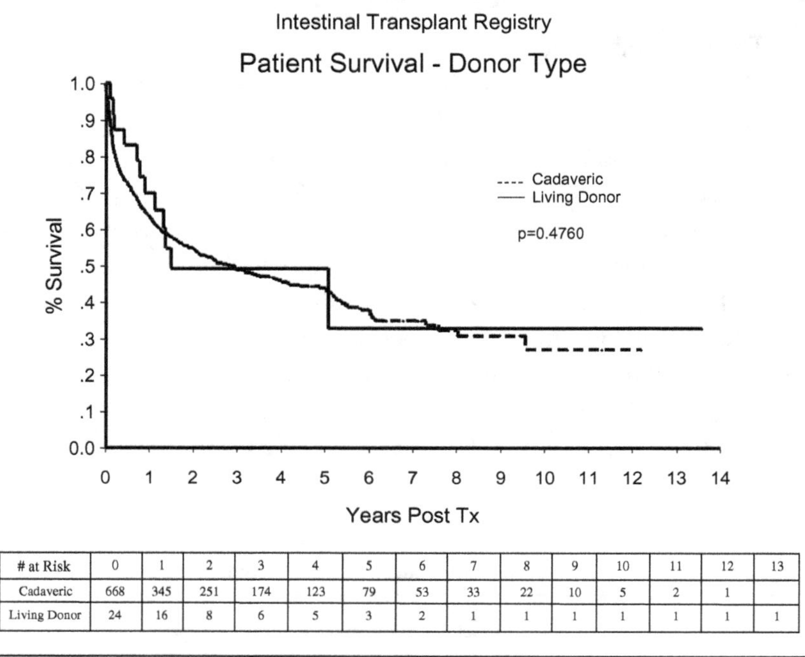

# at Risk	0	1	2	3	4	5	6	7	8	9	10	11	12	13
Cadaveric	668	345	251	174	123	79	53	33	22	10	5	2	1	
Living Donor	24	16	8	6	5	3	2	1	1	1	1	1	1	1

All the living related small bowel recipients have been treated with combination of tacrolimus and steroids, similarly to the current trend in cadaver bowel transplant.

Importantly, the mean waiting time on the list for cadaveric donors in paediatric patients under five years old is 177 days, while for living related small bowel donors it is less than 30 days.

Conclusions

The field of LR-SBTx is a new and exciting one. When a living donor is available, the mortality on the waiting list can be totally avoided, and current results are comparable to those obtained with cadaver donors. Further study, expanded experience and prolonged follow-up are needed to establish the real merits of the procedure.

Acknowledgments

Special thanks to Peter S Knight for editorial assistance and the surgical photographs.

References

1. Starzl TE, Todo S, Tzakis A, *et al.* The many faces of multivisceral transplants. *Surg. Gynecol. Obstet.* 1991:172:335–44.
2. Todo S, Reyes J, Furukawa H, *et al.* Outcome analysis of 71 clinical intestinal transplantations. *Ann. Surg.* 1995;222:270–82.
3. Gruessner RW, Sharp HL. Living-related intestinal transplantation: first report of a standardized surgical technique. *Transplantation* 1997;11:271–4.
4. Pinna AD, Weppler D, Nery J, *et al.* Intestine transplantation at the University of Miami: five years of experience. *Transplant. Proc.* 2000;32:1226–7.
5. Benedetti E, Baum C, Raofi V, *et al.* Living related small bowel transplantation: progressive functional adaptation of the graft. *Transplant. Proc.* 2000; 32(6):1209.
6. Cicalese L, Rastellini C, Sileri P, *et al.* Segmental living related small bowel transplantation in adults. *J. Gastrointest. Surg.* 2001;5(2):168–73.
7. The Intestinal Transplant Registry. Available at: http://www.intestinaltransplant.org/. Accessed 7 January 2002.
8. UNOS Registry. www.unos.org.
9. Jaffe B. Current indications for and prospects of living related intestinal transplantation. *Curr. Opin. Organ Transplant.* 2000;5:290–4.
10. Dudrick SJ, Wilmore DW, Vars HM. Long-term total parenteral nutrition with growth, development and positive nitrogen balance. *Surgery* 1968;169: 134–42.
11. Benedetti E, Baum C, Cicalese L, *et al.* Progressive functional adaptation of segmental bowel graft from living related donor. *Transplantation* 2001;27(7):569–71.
12. Lee RG, Nakamura K, Tsamandas AC, *et al.* Pathology of human intestine transplantation. *Gastroenterology* 1996;110:1820–34.
13. Goulet O, Jan D, Lacaille F, *et al.* Intestinal transplantation in children: results from Paris. Presented at the VII International Small Bowel Transplant Symposium; 12–15 September 2001; Stockholm, Sweden. Abstract 79.

14. Beat SV, McKiernan PJ, Brook GA, *et al.* Ten-years experience of pediatric intestinal transplantation. Presented at the VII International Small bowel Transplant Symposium; 12–15 September 2001; Stockholm, Sweden. Abstract 77.
15. Grant D. International Intestine Transplant Registry Data. www.lhsc.on.ca/itr.;2001. Accessed 31 May 2002.
16. Ghobrial RM, Farmer DG, Amersi F, *et al.* Advances in pediatric liver and intestinal transplantation. *Am. J. Surg.* 2000;180:328–34.
17. Reyes J, Abu-Elmagd K. Small bowel and liver transplantation in children. In *Diseases of the Biliary System in Children.* Ed: DA Kelly. Osney Mead, Oxford: Blackwell Science, Ltd. 1999, pp 313–31.
18. Abu-Elmagd KM, Reyes J, Todo S, *et al.* Clinical intestinal transplantation: new perspectives and immunologic considerations. *J. Am. Coll. Surg.* 1998; 186:512–27.
19. Gupte GL, Mutimer D, Sandhu D, *et al.* Post-transplant lymphoproliferative disease (PTLD) after intestinal transplantation – a single centre experience. Presented at the VII International Small Bowel Transplant Symposium; 12–15 September 2001; Stockholm, Sweden. Abstract 42.
20. Grant DR. Immunosuppression for small bowel transplantation. *Clin. Transplant.* 1991;5:563–7.
21. Abu-Elmagd KM, Reyes J, Fung JJ, *et al.* Clinical intestine transplantation in 1998: Pittsburgh experience. *Acta Gastroenterol. Belg.* 1999;62:244–7.
22. Reyes J, Tzakis AG, Todo S, *et al.* Small bowel and liver/small bowel transplantation in children. *Sem. Pediatr. Surg.* 1993;2:289–300.
23. Reyes J, Bueno J, Kocoshis S, *et al.* Current status of intestinal transplantation in children. *J. Pediatr. Surg.* 1998;33:243–54.
24. Green M, Bueno J, Rowe D, *et al.* Predictive negative value of persistent low Epstein-Barr virus viral load after intestinal transplantation in children. *Transplantation* 2000;70:593–6.
25. Farmer DG, McDiarmid SV, Yersiz H, *et al.* Improved outcome after intestinal transplantation: an eight-year, single-centre experience. *Transplant. Proc.* 2000;32:1233–4.
26. Beath SV, Protheroe SP, Brook GA, *et al.* Early experience of pediatric intestinal transplantation in United Kingdom, 1993 to 1999. *Transplant. Proc.* 2000;32:1225.

27. Nalesnik M, Demetris AJ, Fung JJ, *et al.* Post-transplantation lymphoproliferative disorders. In *Transplantation Clinical Management Vol. 4.* Medscape Transplantation. 2000.
28. Sigurdsson L, Reyes J, Kocoshis SA, *et al.* Bacteremia after intestinal transplantation in children correlates temporally with rejection or gastrointestinal lymphoproliferative disease. *Transplantation* 2000;70:302–5.
29. Reyes J, Selby R, Abu-Elmagd K, *et al.* Intestinal and multiple organ transplantation. In *Textbook of Critical Care.* 4th edn. Eds: WC Shoemaker, SM Ayers, NA Grenvik, PR Holbrook. Philadelphia: WB Saunders Company. 1999, pp 1678–87.

Chapter 6

Living Donor Lobar Lung Transplantation

Hiroshi Date and Nobuyoshi Shimizu

Introduction

Living-donor lobar lung transplantation (LDLLT) was introduced by Starnes and his colleagues for patients who were thought to be too critical to wait for a cadaveric lung transplantation.[1] A single donor was used in the beginning and successful living-donor single lobe transplantation has been reported for a 12-year-old female with bronchopulmonary dysplasia. However, the following experience of single lobe transplantation was not satisfactory.[2] It is for this reason that Starnes' group has developed a bilateral LDLLT in which two healthy donors donate their right or left lower lobes (Fig. 1).[3,4]

Because only two lobes are transplanted, LDLLT seems to be best suited for children and small adults, and has been applied most exclusively to cystic fibrosis.[3] Recently, Starnes' group has expanded indications for LDLLT to include paediatric patients with PPH, bronchiolitis obliterans and adult patients with pulmonary fibrosis.[5] We began to apply the procedure to a wider range of pathophysiology both for paediatric and adult patients.[6] As of 2003, LDLLT has been performed in approximately 200 patients worldwide. This chapter is written on the basis of our initial experience in LDLLT for 23 patients with various lung diseases.

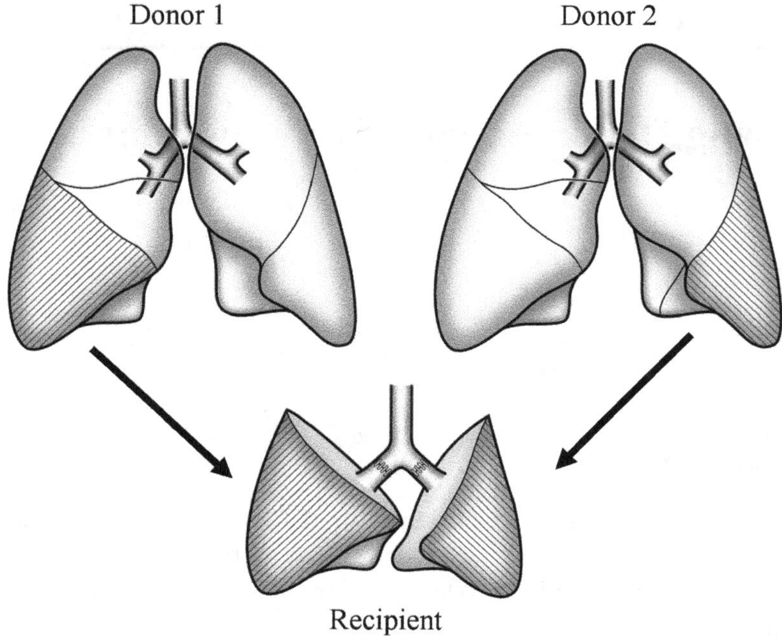

Figure 1: Bilateral living-donor lobar lung transplantation.

Evaluation and Selection in the Donor

Potential donors should be informed about possible perioperative complications and about the permanent loss of their pulmonary function. Although immediate family members (relatives within the second degree or a spouse) have been the only donors in our institution,[6] Starnes' group has accepted extended family members and unrelated individuals.[3] HLA matching is not required for donor selection.

Inclusion criteria for donors are as follows:

- Relatives within the second degree or a spouse
- $20 \leqq \text{Age} \leqq 55$ years
- ABO compatibility
- No significant medical history or active medical problems
- No recent viral infection

- No abnormalities on the echocardiogram
- No abnormalities on the electrocardiogram
- No significant pulmonary pathology on computed tomography on donor side
- Arterial oxygen tension >80 mmHg
- Forced vital capacity, forced expiratory volume in one second >85% of predicted
- No previous thoracic operation on donor side.

Potential donors should be interviewed by two or more physicians with an observer to safeguard against coercion and to ensure donor comprehension of the procedure. The interview should be repeated to provide potential donors multiple opportunities to question, reconsider, or withdraw as a donor. The larger donor is selected for donation of the right lower lobe.

Evaluation and Selection in the Recipient

Patients being considered for LDLLT should meet the criteria for conventional bilateral lung transplantation. The policy of our programme has been to limit LDLLT to critically ill patients who are unlikely to survive the long wait for cadaveric lungs. Controversy exists if LDLLT can be applied to patients already on a ventilator or an extracorporeal membrane oxygenation (ECMO). We have successfully performed LDLLT for a patient with cystic fibrosis who had been on a ventilator for seven weeks.

Size Matching

Appropriate size matching between donor and recipient is important in LDLLT. It is often inevitable to implant small grafts in LDLLT in which only two lobes are implanted. Excessively small grafts may cause high pulmonary artery pressure, resulting in lung edema.[7] A pleural space problem may increase the risk of empyema. Over-expansion of the donor lobes may contribute obstructive physiology by early closure of small airways.[8]

We have previously proposed a formula to estimate the graft forced vital capacity (FVC) based on the donor's measured FVC and the number of pulmonary segments implanted.[6] Given that the right lower lobe consists of five segments, the left lower lobe of four and the whole lung of 19, total FVC of the two grafts is estimated by the following equation:

$$\begin{aligned}&\text{Total FVC of the two grafts}\\&\quad= \text{Measured FVC of the right donor} \times \frac{5}{19}\\&\quad\quad+ \text{Measured FVC of the left donor} \times \frac{4}{19}\end{aligned}$$

When the total FVC of the two grafts is more than 50% of the predicted FVC of the recipient (calculated from a knowledge of height, age and sex), we accept the size disparity regardless of the recipient's diagnosis.

$$\frac{\text{Total FVC of the two grafts}}{\text{Predicted FVC of the recipient}} > 0.5$$

Surgical Technique in the Donor

Epidural catheters for postoperative analgesia are placed routinely the day before the surgery to avoid complications related to heparinization during the donor lobectomies. The recipient and the right-side donor are brought to the separate operating rooms at the same time. The left-side donor is brought to the third operating room 30 minutes later. Three surgical teams are required and they communicate closely to minimize graft ischemic time. After induction of general anaesthesia, donors are intubated with a left-sided double lumen endotracheal tube. Fiberoptic bronchoscopy is performed to determine if lower lobectomy is feasible leaving adequate length for closure on the donor bronchus and length for anastomosis in the recipient.

The donors are placed in the lateral decubitus position and a posterolateral thoracotomy is performed though the fifth intercostal space. Fissures are developed using linear stapling devices. The pericardium surrounding the inferior pulmonary vein is opened circumferentially. Dissection in the fissure is carried out to isolate the pulmonary artery to

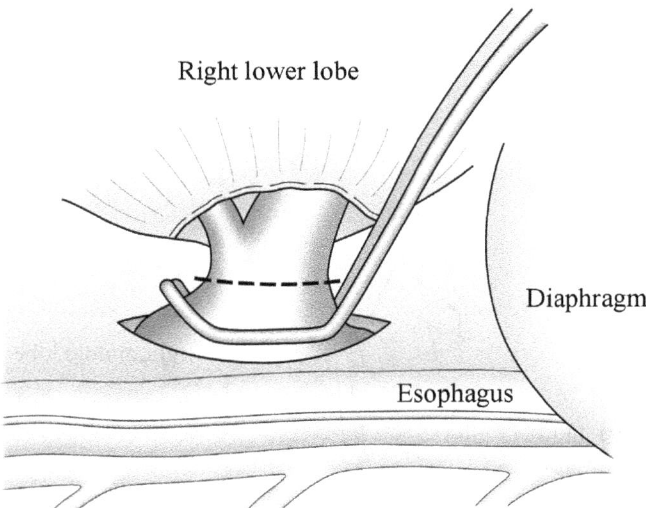

Figure 2: Dissection and division of the right inferior pulmonary vein for donor right lower lobectomy. The pericardium surrounding the inferior pulmonary vein is opened circumferentially. A vascular clamp is placed on the intrapericardial left atrium.

the lower lobe, and to define the anatomy of the pulmonary arteries to the middle lobe in the right-side donor and to the lingular segment in the left-side donor. If the branches of middle lobe artery and lingular artery are small, they are ligated and divided. Intravenous prostaglandin E1 is administered to decrease a systolic blood pressure by 10 to 20 mmHg. Five thousand units of heparin and 500 mg of methylprednisolone are administered intravenously. After placing vascular clamps in appropriate positions, the division of the pulmonary vein (Fig. 2), the pulmonary artery (Fig. 3) and bronchus (Fig. 4) are carried out in this order. Vascular stumps are oversewn with a 5-0 Prolene continuous suture. The bronchial stump is closed with 3-0 Prolene interrupted sutures. Then, each bronchial closure is covered with a pedicled pericardial fat tissue. Heparinization is reversed by administering protamine.

On the back table, the lobes are flushed with 1 L of Euro-Collins solution both antegradely and retrogradely from a bag about 50 cm above the table. Lobes are gently ventilated with room air during the flush.

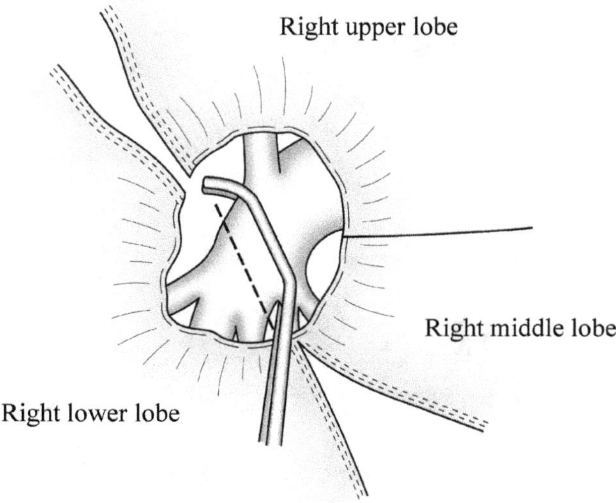

Figure 3: Dissection and division of the pulmonary artery for donor right lower lobectomy.

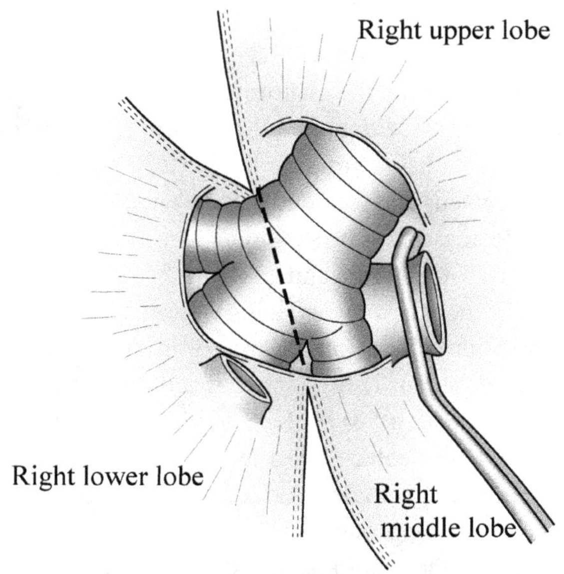

Figure 4: Dissection and division of the right lower bronchus. Great care must be taken to preserve the middle bronchus.

Surgical Technique in the Recipient

Patients are anaesthetized and intubated with a single lumen endotracheal tube in children and with a left-sided double lumen endotracheal tube in adults. A Swan-Ganz catheter is placed. Intraoperative transesophageal echocardiography is employed routinely. The 'clamshell' incision is used and the sternum is transected (Fig. 5). The sternum is notched at the level of transsection by aiming the sternal saw at a 45 degree angle and cutting toward the midpoint to facilitate postoperative sternal adaptation. Pleural and hilar dissection is carried out before heparinization to reduce blood loss. The ascending aorta and the right atrium are cannulated after heparinization and patients are placed on standard cardiopulmonary bypass. After bilateral pneumonectomy, the right lower lobe implantation is performed followed by the left lower lobe implantation. The first implanted right graft is packed in iced saline and slush while the left graft is implanted. The sequence of the recipient anastomosis is the bronchus (Fig. 6), vein (Fig. 7) and artery (Fig. 8). The bronchial anastomosis is begun with a running 4-0 polydioxanone suture for membranous portion and completed with simple interrupted sutures for cartilaginous portion. We use end-to-end anastomosis

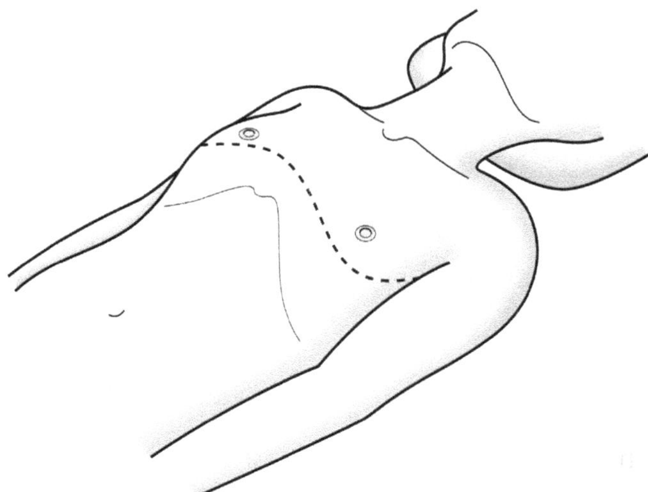

Figure 5: The recipient is placed in a spine position and the 'clamshell' incision is used.

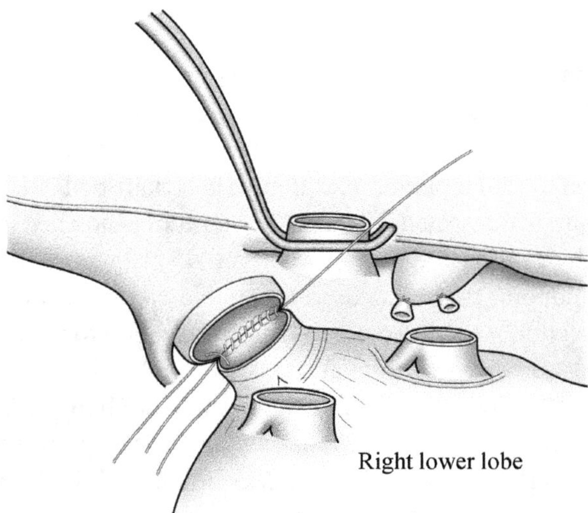

Figure 6: A right bronchial anastomosis. The membranous portion is anastomosed with a running 4-0 polydioxanone suture.

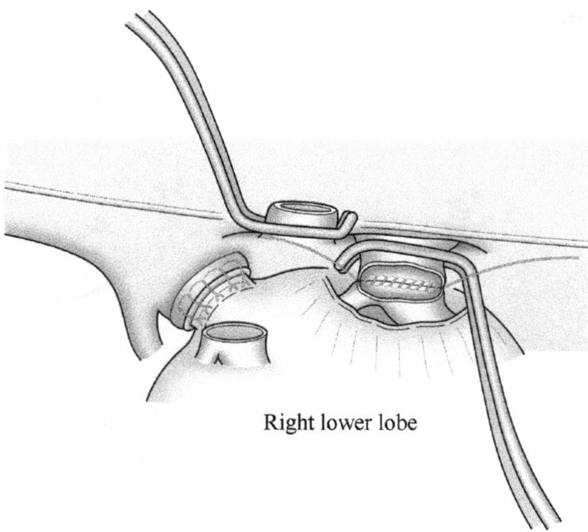

Figure 7: The bronchial anastomosis is completed with simple interrupted sutures for cartilaginous portion. The venous anastomosis is conducted between the donor right inferior pulmonary vein and the recipient right superior pulmonary vein using a 6-0 Prolene continuous suture.

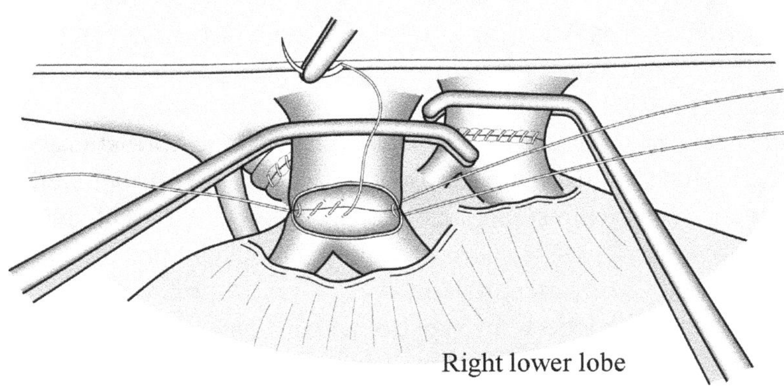

Figure 8: The pulmonary artery anastomosis is performed using a running 6-0 Prolene suture interrupted at either end.

when the bronchial size is equivalent, and use telescoping technique when the discrepancy in bronchial size is obvious. The bronchial wrapping is not employed except for the patients on high-dose steroid therapy. Peribronchial connective tissue or pedicled pericardial fat tissue is used to cover the bronchial anastomosis if necessary. Just before completing the bilateral implantations, 500 mg to 1 g of methylprednisolone is given intravenously and nitric oxide inhalation is initiated at 20 ppm. After both lungs are reperfused and ventilated, cardiopulmonary bypass is gradually weaned and then removed. All blood accumulated in the chest cavity during the operation is discarded to avoid infection. Two chest tubes are placed in each chest cavity and the chest is closed in the standard fashion.

At the conclusion of the operation, a nasal feeding tube is inserted to the proximal jejunum under the fluoroscope. The feeding tube is very useful for drug delivery and for enteral nutrition.

Complications in the Donor

There has been a relatively low incidence of donor morbidity in our experience and all donors have returned to their previous lifestyles. However, serious complications, such as bronchial fistula, pulmonary embolism, have been reported.[9] No mortality has been reported.

Among the 45 donors in our centre, two donors required re-thoracotomy due to bleeding from chest wall; however, none of the patients required transfusion. Three donors developed middle lobe pneumonia associated with mild bronchial stricture. They were successfully treated with antibiotics and did not require bronchial dilatation. Atrial fibrillation, wound infection, cholecystitis and haemosputum were also seen but were conservatively treated with symptomatic improvement. One right-side donor required reconstruction of the middle lobe bronchus after the bronchus intermedius was inadvertently divided.

Although donor lobectomy is performed on young healthy individuals, the incidence of perioperative complications related to donor lobectomy may be higher than that of standard lobectomy for lung cancer.[9] Donor lobectomy should be performed only by well-experienced thoracic surgeons.

Complications in the Recipient

The operative morbidity of the recipients is very high; therefore meticulous postoperative management is mandatory.

We have encountered various operative complications and some of them were unique to LDLLT. Lung edema was the most common complication. Knowing that the graft ischemic time was short in this procedure, the high incidence of lung edema must be related to the small grafts implanted. Of note was that half of primary pulmonary hypertension (PPH) patients required re-intubation due to lung edema associated with left ventricular failure on day 5–14, soon after they were extubated. Life threatening massive haemoptysis was encountered in one patient, which was successfully treated with ECMO.[10] Bronchoscopic examination demonstrated normal bronchial healing and chest radiography revealed pulmonary haemorrhages in the right graft. Although the cause of the bleeding was unknown, it could be related to increased blood flow in the small grafts implanted. Transient haemolytic anaemia occurred in one patient receiving LDLLT with a minor ABO mismatch.[11] The patient was group A and received lobes from donors with group O. Donor-derived lymphocytes from group O lungs produced anti-A antibody and caused haemolytic anaemia between ten to 21 days after transplantation.

The patient was successfully treated with transfusion of group O red cells without developing renal dysfunction.

In the other centres with a large percentage of cystic fibrosis patients among recipients, infection has consistently been the major cause of mortality.[12] There were no airway complications in the 45 bronchial anastomoses in our experience.

Protocols of Immunosuppression

Postoperative immunosuppression is a triple drug therapy consisting of cyclosporine (CSA) or tacrolimus (FK), azathioprine (AZA) or mycophenolate mofetil (MMF), and corticosteroids. Induction therapy with monoclonal or polyclonal antibodies is not used.

The combination of CSA + AZA + steroid is chosen for patients with infectious lung diseases and paediatric patients. The combination of FK + MMF + steroid is chosen for patients with non-infectious lung diseases.

CSA (100 mg) or FK (2 mg) delivery begins during the first few post-operative hours via the nasal feeding tube inserted to the proximal jejunum. The dosage is adjusted to maintain trough levels in the target range listed in Table 1. These drugs often induce a significant increase in serum creatinine, necessitating a reduction in their dosage.

AZA (2 mg/kg) or MMF (500 mg) is given orally before operation and then given via the nasal feeding tube post-transplant. The dose must be adjusted to maintain while blood cell count in excess of 3,500. MMF often causes significant diarrhoea, necessitating the dose reduction.

We have adopted the use of moderate dose corticosteroids during the early postoperative period. Intravenous administration of methylprednisolone is used before reperfusion and during the first three days. Then we initiate prednisone via the nasal feeding tube as summarized in Table 1.

Detection and Management of Acute Rejection

In cadaveric lung transplantation, transbronchial lung biopsy offers a safe and accurate means of diagnosis of acute rejection and has emerged as the procedure of choice.[13] However, the risk of pneumothorax and

Table 1: Okayama University triple-drug immunosuppressive protocol for living-donor lobar lung transplantation.

Cyclosporine (Neoral)			
Pre-transplant	None		
Post-transplant	Dosage adjusted to maintain trough level at	3 months post-transplant	250–350 ng/dl
		6 months post-transplant	200–300 ng/dl
		12 months post-transplant	150–250 ng/dl
Tacrolimus (Prograf)			
Pre-transplant	None		
Post-transplant	Dosages adjusted to maintain trough level at	3 months post-transplant	10–20 ng/dl
		6 months post-transplant	10–15 ng/dl
		12 months post-transplant	8–12 ng/dl
Azathioprine (Imuran)			
Pre-transplant	2 mg/kg		
Post-transplant	2 mg/kg		
Mycophenolate mofetil (Cellcept)			
Pre-transplant	500 mg		
Post-transplant	500–1,000 mg twice daily		
Corticosteroids			
Before reperfusion		Methylprednisolone (iv)	1,000 mg
Post-transplant	3 days post-transplant	Methylprednisolone (iv)	125 mg per day
	6 months post-transplant	Prednisone (oral)	0.4 mg/kg per day
	12 months post-transplant	Prednisone (oral)	0.2 mg/kg per two days

bleeding by transbronchial lung biopsy may be higher in LDLLT because small grafts are receiving high blood flow. It is for this reason that we judge acute rejection on the basis of radiographic and clinical findings. Early acute rejection episodes are characterized by dyspnoea, low grade fever, leukocytosis, hypoxaemia and diffuse interstitial infiltrate on chest radiographs. Because two lobes are donated by different donors, acute rejection is usually seen unilaterally. A trial bolus dose of methylprednisolone 500 mg is administered and various clinical signs are carefully observed. If acute rejection is indeed the problem, two additional daily bolus doses of methylprednisolone are given. If acute rejection is encountered more than three times, CSA + AZA is switched to FK + MMF. When all these treatments fail, OKT3 is used (Fig. 9).

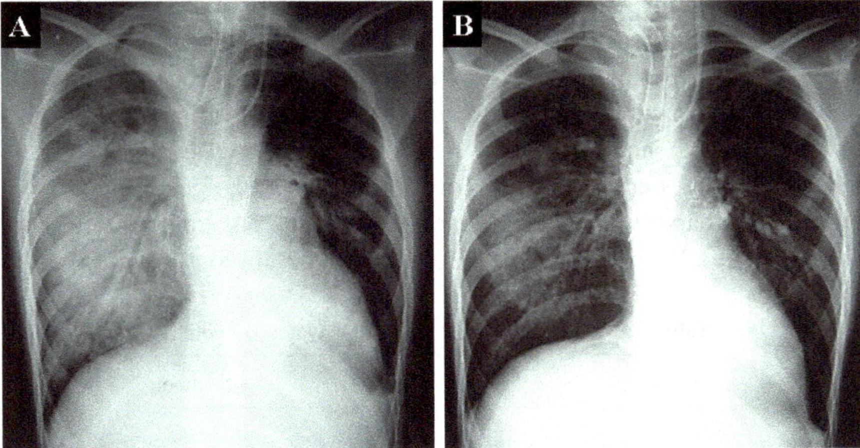

Figure 9: Acute rejection after living-donor lobar lung transplantation. The patient was a 13-year-old female with primary pulmonary hypertension. Acute rejection occurred three times during the first month and was treated with bolus injection of methylprednisolone. She developed the fourth acute rejection in the right graft on day 44 (A) and OKT3 was used. Dramatic improvement was shown two days after OKT3 treatment (B).

Postoperative management

The patient is kept intubated at a positive end-expiratory pressure of 5 cm H_2O for at least three days to maintain optimal expansion of the small lobes implanted. The suction of the chest drainage tubes starts at 10 cm H_2O and gradually decreases to water seal in a couple of days. Fibre-optic bronchoscopy is performed every 12 hours while intubated to assess donor airway viability and to suction any retained secretions. An intensive program of chest physiotherapy is given every four hours and bedside postoperative pulmonary rehabilitation is initiated as soon as possible. Cytomegalovirus prophylaxis with ganciclovir is given to all recipients for the first three months.

Results After Living-Donor Lobar Lung Transplantation

Table 2 lists the preoperative diagnoses of the 23 patients who have undergone LDLLT at Okayama University Hospital from October 1998 through June 2003. Diagnoses included various lung diseases including hypertensive (PPH[14,15] Eisenmenger's syndrome), obstructive (bronchiolitis obliterans[16] lymphangioleiomyomatosis), restrictive (idiopathic interstitial pneumonia) and infectious (bronchiectasis[17] cystic fibrosis) lung diseases. There were 18 females and five males with ages ranging from eight to 53 years (average 28.4 years). Five of the patients were children and 18 were adults. The height ranged from 122 cm to 164 cm (average

Table 2: Diagnoses for LDLLT at Okayama University.

Diagnoses	Number
Primary pulmonary hypertension	9
Idiopathic interstitial pneumonia	4
Bronchiolitis obliterans	3
Bronchiectasis	3
Lymphangioleiomyomatosis	2
Cystic fibrosis	1
Eisenmenger's syndrome	1
Total	23

LDLLT = Living-donor lobar lung transplantation.

151.5 cm) and the weight ranged from 20.0 kg to 60.2 kg (average 39.2 kg). All patients were dependent on continuous oxygen inhalation. Ten patients were steroid-dependent. All nine patients with PPH were on high-dose intravenous epoprostenol (average, 89.0 ng/kg/min) and inotropic therapy. Four patients were ventilator-dependent for two to seven weeks. Five other patients were about to be intubated and required a non-invasive positive pressure ventilator. Eight patients received LDLLT on an emergency basis. Bilateral LDLLT was performed in 22 patients and right single LDLLT was performed for a 10-year-old boy with PPH[15] because his mother was the only available donor.

Among the 45 living-donors, 12 were the mothers of recipients, 11 were brothers, nine were fathers, six were sisters, four were husbands, two were daughters and one was a son. The average height and weight of the right-side donor were 169.4 cm and 70.6 kg, and those of the left-side donor were 160.5 cm and 59.0 kg, respectively. The total FVC of the two grafts was estimated to range from 51.4% to 103.0% (average 66.5%) of the predicted FVC of the recipient.

Thirteen patients received an ABO-identical LDLLT and ten patients received LDLLT with a minor ABO mismatch.

In six patients, partial cardiopulmonary bypass was initiated using the femoral vessels under local anaesthesia because of their unstable preoperative condition. Then, they were anaesthetized and intubated. Cardiopulmonary bypass was successfully removed from all the 23 patients at the end of the procedure. The systolic pulmonary artery pressure was 36.9 ± 1.7 mmHg immediately after the bypass was stopped. The ischemic time of the right graft was 152 ± 7 minutes and that of the left graft was 109 ± 6 minutes.

During the fist month, no infection was encountered and acute rejection occurred 1.5 episodes/patient on average.

For the 23 recipients, duration of mechanical ventilation required was 9.3 ± 1.7 days, ICU stay was 23.1 ± 3.3 days and hospital stay was 61.0 ± 4.3 days. Although their FVC (1,327 ± 78 ml, 50.2% of predicted) was limited at discharge, arterial oxygen tension on room air (98.5 ± 1.8 mmHg) and systolic pulmonary artery pressure (24.8 ± 1.6 mmHg) were excellent. FVC improved gradually and reached 1894 ± 99 ml, 67.4% of predicted, at one year. Their six-minute walking distance also increased gradually during the first year. The recipient's FVC measured at six months (1,813 ± 86 ml) was correlated well with the graft FVC (1,803 ± 70 ml) estimated based on the donor's measured FVC ($r = 0.802$, $p = 0.00098$).[18] There were three recipients (13%) who developed bronchiolitis obliterans syndrome (BOS) after LDLLT.

The dramatic changes in chest X-ray findings were demonstrated in various lung diseases (Figs. 10–12).

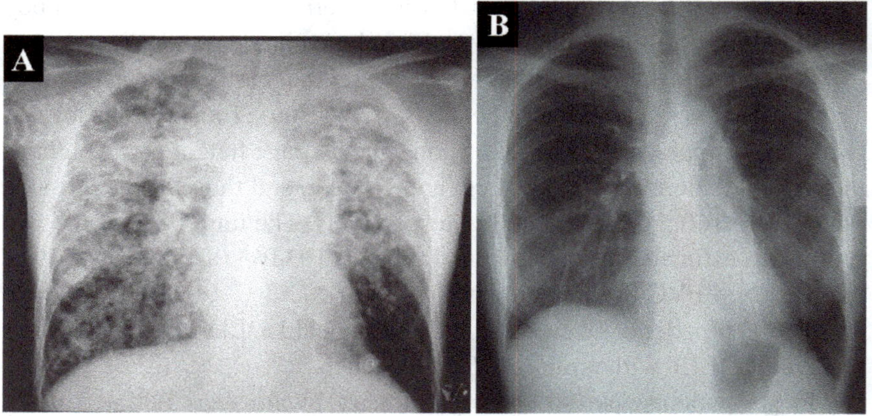

Figure 10: A 24-year-old female with bronchiectasis associated with primary ciliary dyskinesia. (A) Pre-transplant and (B) after receiving LDLLT.

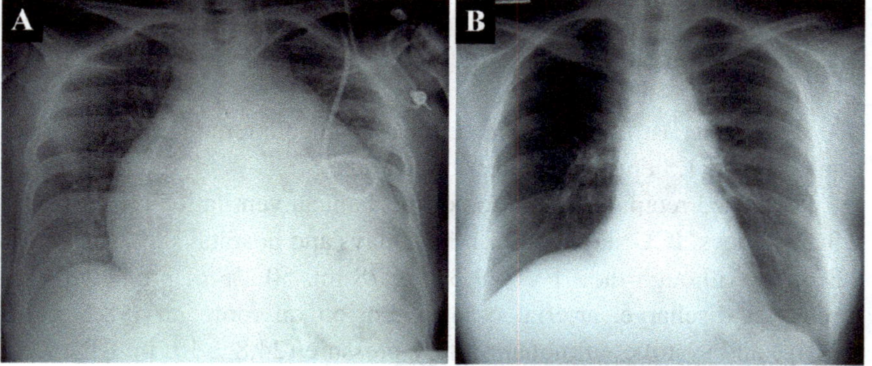

Figure 11: A 27-year-old female with primary pulmonary hypertension. (A) Pre-transplant and (B) after receiving LDLLT.

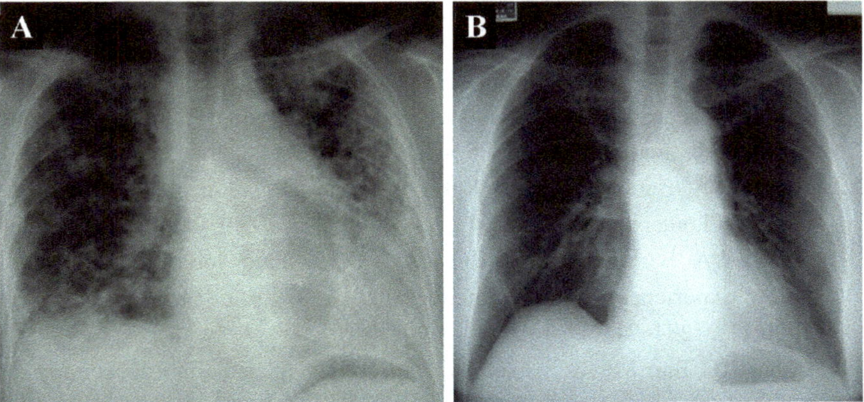

Figure 12: A 53-year-old female with idiopathic interstitial pneumonia. (A) Pre-transplant and (B) after receiving LDLLT.

At the time of final data analysis in July 2003, all the 23 recipients are alive with a follow-up period of one to 57 months. All donors have returned to their previous lifestyles during the observation period.

Conclusion

LDLLT is a new and evolving option for patients with end-stage lung disease. Although our experience in LDLLT is still limited in numbers (n = 23) and in observation period (1–57 months), the 100% successful rate is very encouraging. Meticulous perioperative management, including inhaled nitric oxide, frequent bronchoscopy, an intensive program of chest physiotherapy and routine intubation for at least three days, is very important. We believe that the 'small but perfect graft' is a great advantage in this procedure.

In summary, LDLLT can be applied to various end-stage lung diseases including restrictive, obstructive, infectious and hypertensive lung diseases both for paediatric and adult patients. It offers an alternative to cadaveric lung transplant that results in equivalent or better survival and morbidity.

References

1. Starnes VA, Lewiston NJ, Luikart H, *et al.* Current trends in lung transplantation: lobar transplantation and expanded use of single lungs. *J. Thorac. Cardiovasc. Surg.* 1992;104:1060–8.
2. Starnes VA, Barr ML, Cohen RG. Lobar transplantation: indications, technique, and outcome. *J. Thorac. Cardiovasc. Surg.* 1994;108:403–11.
3. Starnes VA, Barr ML, Cohen RG, *et al.* Living-donor lobar lung transplantation experience: intermediate results. *J. Thorac. Cardiovasc. Surg.* 1996;112:1284–91.
4. Cohen RG, Barr ML, Schenkel FA, *et al.* Living-related donor lobectomy for bilateral lobar transplantation in patients with cystic fibrosis. *Ann. Thorac. Surg.* 1994;57:1423–8.
5. Starnes VA, Barr ML, Schenkel FA, *et al.* Experience with living-donor lobar transplantation for indications other than cystic fibrosis. *J. Thorac. Cardiovasc. Surg.* 1997;114:917–22.
6. Date H, Aoe M, Nagahiro I, *et al.* Living-donor lobar lung transplantation for various lung diseases. *J. Thorac. Cardiovasc. Surg.* 2003;126:476–81.
7. Fujita T, Date H, Ueda K, *et al.* Experimental study on size matching in a canine living-donor lobar lung transplant model. *J. Thorac. Cardiovasc. Surg.* 2002;123:104–9.
8. Haddy SM, Bremner RM, Moore-Jefferies EW, *et al.* Hyperinflation resulting in hemodynamic collapse following living-donor lobar transplantation. *Anesthesiology* 2002;95:1315–7.
9. Battafarano RJ, Anderson RC, Meyers BF, *et al.* Perioperative complications after living-donor lobectomy. *J. Thorac. Cardiovasc. Surg.* 2000;120:909–15.
10. Kotani K, Ichiba S, Andou M, *et al.* Extracorporeal membrane oxygenation with nafamostat mesilate as an anticoagulant for massive pulmonary hemorrhage after living-donor lobar lung transplantation. *J. Thorac. Cardiovasc. Surg.* 2002;124:626–7.
11. Sano Y, Aoe M, Date H, *et al.* Minor ABO-incompatible living-related lung transplantation. *Transplant. Proc.* 2002;34:2807–9.
12. Barr ML, Baker CJ, Schenkel FA, *et al.* Living-donor lung transplantation: selection, technique and outcome. *Transplant. Proc.* 2001;33:3527–32.
13. Trulock EP, Ettinger NA, Brunt EM, *et al.* The role of transbronchial lung biopsy in the treatment of lung transplant recipients: an analysis of 200 consecutive procedures. *Chest* 1992;102:1049–54.

14. Date H, Nagahiro I, Aoe M, *et al.* Living-donor lobar lung transplantation for primary pulmonary hypertension in an adult. *J. Thorac. Cardiovasc. Surg.* 2001;122:817–8.
15. Date H, Sano Y, Aoe M, *et al.* Living-donor single lobe lung transplantation for primary pulmonary hypertension in a child. *J. Thorac. Cardiovasc. Surg.* 2002;123:1211–3.
16. Date H, Sano Y, Aoe M, *et al.* Living-donor lobar lung transplantation for bronchiolitis obliterans after Stevens-Johnson syndrome. *J. Thorac. Cardiovasc. Surg.* 2002;123:389–91.
17. Date H, Yamashita M, Nagahiro I, *et al.* Living-donor lobar lung transplantation for primary ciliary dyskinesia. *Ann. Thorac. Surg.* 2001;71:2008–9.
18. Date H, Aoe M, Nagahiro I, *et al.* How to predict forced vital capacity after living-donor lobar lung transplantation. *J. Heart Lung Transplant.* 2004;23:547–51.

Chapter 7

Allogeneic Haemopoietic Stem Cell Transplantation

Eduardo Olavarria

Introduction

The field of allogeneic haemopoietic stem cell transplantation (HSCT) and increasingly the use of cellular therapy have continued to evolve since their origins in the early 1900s. Results are improving constantly mainly due to a combination of better understanding of the underlying biological background and major advances in supportive care. New diseases and indications have been developed and with the advent of reduced toxicity conditioning, this treatment modality has been extended to older patients and to patients who in previous times would have been considered ineligible for transplantation.

With increasing knowledge of the immunobiology of allogeneic transplantation and the development of more precise techniques for tissue typing and characterization of the human histocompatibility genes, the use of alternative donors such as mismatched family members, matched or mismatched unrelated volunteers or cord blood stem cells has become widely accepted.

Historical background

In the first half of the 20th century, there had been attempts to use bone marrow tissue for its therapeutic effects in anaemia and leukaemia by oral, intramuscular or intravenous routes.[1,2] In 1922, a Danish investigator, Fabriciuos Moeller, noted that guinea pigs, whose legs were protected from total body lethal irradiation, were able to survive this procedure and did not develop thrombocytopenia a haemorrhagic diathesis.[3] His findings were ignored for some years, until the mid-1950s, when Jacobson showed that lethally irradiated mice could be protected by intraperitoneal injection of spleen cells (a haematopoietic organ in the mouse) or intravenous infusion of bone marrow.[4]

Although initial consideration was given to a humoral factor, by the end of the decade, several reports had shown that the protection was due to the presence of donor cells in the bone marrow of the irradiated mice.[1,5,6] Ford *et al.* designated an animal that carried a mixture of its own and foreign haematopoietic cells as a radiation chimera.[7]

During the first years of experimental marrow transplantation, the emphasis was on radiation protection. However, subsequent studies focusing on the ultimate fate of the transplanted animals showed that many animals initially survived but later died of severe diarrhoea, weight loss and skin lesions.[1,8] These observations rapidly led to the description of a 'secondary disease' initially termed runting syndrome.[9] This runt disease was in fact graft versus host disease (GVHD) and by the late 1960s it was clear that this was caused by the lymphocytes in the infused graft and that it was mediated by alloantigens present in the host but absent in the donor.[8,9]

The next step was the discovery of tolerance induced by marrow transplantation. Main and Prehn reported that mice surviving allogeneic marrow transplantation following total body irradiation (TBI) were able to permanently accept skin grafts from the original donor strain.[10] This was also demonstrated for xenografts using mice and rats.[11] Later on animal models of malignant disease were produced and studies showed that TBI followed by infusion of bone marrow cells was able to produce long-term cure, although most animals still perished following the development of GVHD. Some studies suggested that lymphohaemopoietic tumours were more susceptible to the antitumour effect than sarcomas and carcinomas, perhaps due to the relative richness of transplantation alloantigens in these malignancies.

Although the major histocompatibility complex (MHC) had been known since the late 1930s, it was not until the late 1960s and early 1970s that the concept of histocompatibility was fully established in allogeneic haemopoietic cell transplantation. However, in 1957 Thomas reported that large amounts of human marrow cells could be infused safely and describe the first (albeit transient) marrow graft in patients affected of acute leukaemia.[12] In 1959 Mathé and co-workers attempted to treat six patients who had been exposed to high doses of radiation during an accident in Vinca, Serbia.[13] Several groups in the USA and Europe started bone marrow transplant programmes with disappointing results. Most of these patients had end-stage acute leukaemia, were frequently severely infected at the time of transplant and died before proper assessment could be carried out. The following decade was fraught with frustration, and when patients survived the initial phase of the transplant with apparently successful engraftment of the donor marrow cells, they often died of severe GVHD or late infections. It is worth mentioning that many of these transplants were performed without any tissue typing or using techniques that were found later to be unreliable.

In 1977 the Seattle group reported the results of human leukocyte antigen (HLA) identical sibling bone marrow transplants in 100 patients with end-stage acute leukaemia.[14] This classic study confirmed the curative potential of marrow transplantation in acute leukaemia with 13 very long-term disease-free survivors. However, the initial enthusiasm about these remarkable results was tempered by the actuarial relapse rate of nearly 70% and the high incidence of transplant-related deaths.[14] The authors hypothesized that transplants performed in early remission stages would fare better and in 1979 they reported that of 19 patients transplanted from HLA identical siblings in first complete remission of their acute leukaemia, ten were alive and leukaemia free.[15] It is generally accepted that the modern era of bone marrow transplantation began in the 1970s when reliable HLA typing was available and when patients with acute leukaemia were transplanted in early remission.

Only 30–40% of patients who are candidates for bone marrow transplantation will have an HLA identical sibling. There are now well over 13 million bone marrow volunteer donors in the different international registries (Fig. 1). As always, the use of alternative donors was marked by advances in molecular typing of the different HLA genes and the improvement in the management of post-transplant complications. Currently,

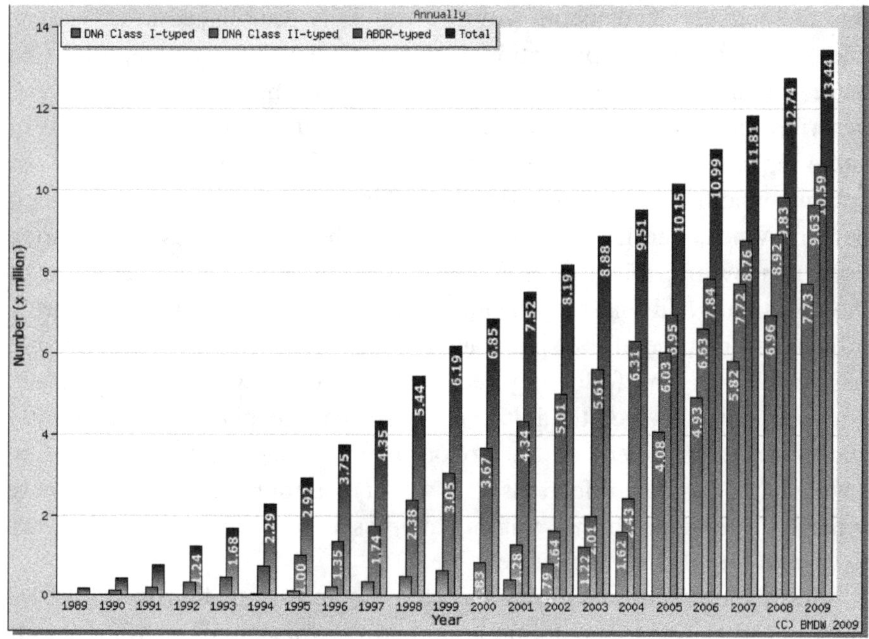

Figure 1: Number of unrelated stem cell donors and cord blood units in the international registries since the year 1989.

Source: http://www.bmdw.org.

more than 15,000 allogeneic stem cell transplants are carried out each year worldwide demonstrating the important role that this treatment modality plays in the management of haematological malignancies.

The Role of HLA in HSCT

Tissue compatibility is determined by genes of the major histocompatibility complex (MHC), known as the HLA system in man, which are clustered on the short arm of chromosome 6. The HLA region is a multigenic system that encodes structurally homologous cell surface glycoproteins characterized by a high degree of allelic polymorphism within human populations. Immune responses against incompatible HLA Ag represent a major barrier to HSCT. The accuracy of histocompatibility testing and matching criteria will therefore have important consequences on graft outcome. This is particularly true in the case of transplantation with HSC from unrelated donors (UD), where serologically hidden incompatibilities may account for the increased rate of post-transplant complications.

The homologous HLA class I (HLA-A, -B, -C) and class II (HLA-DR, -DQ, -DP) antigens are codominantly expressed and differ in their structure, tissue distribution and characteristics in peptide presentation to T-cells.[16] The biological function of HLA molecules is to present peptide Ag to T-cells, thereby playing a key role in T-cell-mediated adaptive immunity.

HLA class I molecules are expressed on most nucleated cells. They are composed of an alpha-chain (encoded in the MHC) non-covalently associated with Beta-2-microglobulin (encoded on chromosome 15). Peptides (usually of 8–10 aminoacids) presented by class I molecules are derived from proteolytic degradation of cytoplasmic proteins by the proteasome, transported across the endoplasmic reticulum where they bind to class I Ag. Pathogen-derived peptides presented to class I Ag are usually recognized by CD8+ CTL.[16] HLA class II Ag are expressed on a subset of cells of the immune system comprising dendritic cells, B-cells, activated T-cells, macrophages, collectively referred to as Ag presenting cells (APC). They are heterodimers composed of two membrane-bound chains that are encoded by two genes that co-localize in the MHC. The peptide-binding pocket is formed by the most distal domains of the two chains. Extracellular Ag internalized by endocytosis/phagocytosis are degraded in an endocytic compartment into peptides of 10–30 amino acids that bind class II molecules. HLA class II-peptide complexes expressed on the membrane are usually recognized by CD4+ T-helper cells.[16]

The HLA system comprises 12 genes located on a 3.6 Mb segment of the short arm of chromosome 6. Three HLA class I genes (A, B, C) encode respectively for the heavy chains of HLA-A, -B and -C antigens. HLA class II Ag (DR, DQ, DP) are heterodimers encoded by an alpha-chain and a beta-chain gene (e.g. DRA/DRB1 or DQA1/DQB1) that co-localize at the centromeric part of the MHC.[16,17] The HLA-DR subregion presents an additional complexity level since a second DRB gene may be present, i.e. DRB3 in DR11/DR12/DR13/DR14/DR17/DR18 haplotypes, DRB4 in

DR4/DR7/DR9 haplotypes, and DRB5 in DR15/DR16 haplotype. Because of the codominant expression of HLA genes, a heterozygous individual may express up to 12 different HLA Ag.

In the early 1990s the role of HLA matching was hampered by the poor resolution achieved by HLA typing, particularly for HLA class I alleles. Based on high-resolution typing methods more recent studies[18–22] reached the almost general consensus that allele-level matching does improve transplant outcome. However the relative importance of individual loci still remains under investigation.

Graft failure: The role of HLA-A/B/C/DR mismatches has been shown by several studies. The total number of disparities influences the risk of graft failure.[18–20] A comparison of serological versus allele class I mismatches in CML patients suggested that qualitative differences may influence the risk of graft failure, with a higher risk in serotype-mismatched patients.[19]

Graft versus host disease (GVHD): Multiple class I, or class II, or combined class I and II mismatches correlated with an increased risk of GVHD.[19] In the Japanese Marrow Donor Program (JMDP) study[20] HLA-A/B/C/DRB1 mismatches were found to be significant risk factors for grades III–IV acute GVHD, whereas the American National Marrow Donor Program (NMDP) data revealed a DRB1 effect with no contribution of HLA-DQ/DP[21] or HLA-B/C[22] mismatches. A few studies reported an association of HLA-DP disparities with an increased rate of acute GVHD.

Survival: HLA-A/B/C/DRB1, but not DQ/DP mismatches decreased survival in the NMDP study,[21,22] whereas in the JMDP study only A/B/DRB1 disparities were associated with mortality.[20] In chronic myeloid leukaemia (CML) patients from the Seattle study a single class II mismatch was well tolerated whereas single class I or multiple mismatches were associated with lower survival.[18,19] Differences between studies may involve selection criteria of each transplant centre, patients age or other pre-transplant risk factors, experience in treating GVHD, as well as the relevance of the GvL effect in CML patients. In the largest cohort of CML patients studied so far,[23] HLA-AB-serology/DRB1-allele 'matched' unrelated HSCT were compared to matched sibling donor HSCT patients. Multivariate analysis revealed SRV rates lower than five-years after 'matched' unrelated versus matched sibling donor HSCT. Such decreased survival possibly results, at least in part, from the presence of undisclosed HLA-A/B/C allele mismatches in the so-called 'matched' unrelated donors.

Sources and Procurement of Allogeneic Haematopoietic Stem Cells

The preferred source of progenitor cells for HSCT has changed over the years. Traditionally, cells were harvested from the iliac crests under general anaesthesia, but recently G-CSF mobilized peripheral blood (PB) has been increasingly used. Unmanipulated cord blood (CB) cells collected and cryopreserved at birth have been used both in related and unrelated HLA matched and mismatched allogeneic transplants in children and more recently in adults. It has become evident that there are many quantitative and qualitative differences between these cell sources (Table 1).

In 1995, three pivotal studies demonstrated the safety and feasibility of using G-CSF mobilized PB allografts.[24] Patients experienced prompt

Table 1: Advantages and disadvantages in the search and identification process of BM and CB unrelated donor.

	Bone marrow	Cord blood
Information on A+B+DRB1(DNA) type	16–56%	50–80%
Median search time	3–6 months	<1 month
Donors identified but not available	30%	<1%
Rare haplotypes represented	2%	29%
Major limiting factors to graft acquisition	HLA match	Cell dose
Ease of rearranging date of cell infusion	Difficult	Easy
Potential for second HSC graft or DLI	Yes	No from the same donor
Potential — for viral transmission	Yes	No
— for congenital diseases	No	Yes
Risk to donor	Yes	No

engraftment with an incidence of GVHD similar to that of bone marrow (BM) recipients. In addition, no serious short-term complications of G-CSF mobilized PB harvesting were observed in the donors.[24–26] Direct comparison of PB and BM in allogeneic sibling donor transplantation has been reported in at least eight randomized trials.[25–32] Most of them did not show a survival benefit (Table 2). The incidence of acute GVHD was similar in all but one of the studies, but an increase (statistically significant or a trend) in the incidence of overall and extensive chronic GVHD was demonstrated in recipients of PBSC allografts. The magnitude of this observation and its effect on relapse, survival and recipient quality of life is less clear. In unrelated transplant recipients, matched cohort comparisons of UD, BMT and PBSCT reported faster haematological recovery among PB recipients with no difference in either acute GVHD or chronic GVHD.

While results of randomized studies are pending, the use of PB allografts in UD HSCT has varied among transplant centres and countries. Some registries of unrelated marrow donors have permitted the collection of allografts from the PB whereas others have not. Transplant centres may request a PB or a BM graft but the collection centre and wishes of

Table 2: Relapse incidence (RI) and survival after allo-PBSCT compared to allo-BMT in different randomized studies.

Reference	Source	n	RI		Survival
Bensinger	BM	91	25%	54%	Early status: 72% vs 75% p = ns
	PBSC	81	14%	66%	Advanced: 33% vs 57%, p = .04
			p = 0.04	p = .06	
Blaise	BM	52		65%	
	PBSC	48	ns	67% p = ns	
Heldal	BM	30			
	PBSC	28	ns	p = ns	
Powles	BM	19	0%	63%	
	PBSC	18	37%	70% p = ns	
Schmitz	BM	166			
	PBSC	163	ns	ns	
Vigoritto	BM	19			
	PBSC	18	ns	ns	

the donor also determine which product is ultimately collected. Because of the absence of definitive data comparing both sources of cells, there is no indication to prefer either source of cells except perhaps in patients with advanced disease where chronic GVHD and subsequent GvL might decrease relapse and improve survival, or in a situation where a high number of cells is necessary for engraftment, for example after non-myeloablative conditioning or if TCD is planned for a HLA mismatched transplant.

Principles of Conditioning Regimens

The diversity of today's conditioning regimens is based on its historical development (Table 3). The effects of total body irradiation (TBI) on BM provided a concept for BMT experiments in animals and man. It became possible to eliminate a diseased haematopoietic system without causing irreversible damage of other organs. TBI was intended to be an equivalent to surgical removal in solid organ transplantation. Therefore the term 'to condition' meant the preparation of the recipient to accept a new organ in place of the diseased haematopoietic system.[33]

There are three main objectives: space-making, immunosuppression and disease eradication. The first of these is a somewhat controversial concept which originated from the belief that immature progenitor cells occupy defined niches within the marrow stroma in order to obtain the necessary support for proliferation and differentiation. To allow access to these niches, existing host stem cell cells must be eradicated in order for donor engraftment to occur. Immunosuppression is required to prevent rejection of the incoming donor cells by residual host haematopoiesis. The probability of rejection is increased in situations of increasing HLA-disparity, e.g. volunteer UD and family mismatched transplants or in situations where the recipient has been 'pre-sensitized' by the administration of multiple blood products prior to HSCT. It is also increased in T-cell depleted (TCD) HSCT. On the other hand, rejection (and relapse) is decreased by reduced GVHD prophylaxis, high stem cell dose and high T-cell dose. The ultimate role of the conditioning regimen is long-term disease control. This is a clear objective in the haematological malignancies, but it is also of vital importance in diseases characterized by

Table 3: Common conditioning regimens.

Regimen	Total dose	Daily dose	Administration	Days
Conventional "old" regimens				
Cy/TBI				
Cyclosphosphamide	120 mg/kg	60 mg/kg	IV in 1 hour	-6, -5
Total body irradiation	12–14.4 Gy	2–2.4 Gy (2x/day)		-3, -2, -1
Bu/Cy				
Busulfan	16 mg/kg	4 mg/kg	p.o. q 6 hour	-9, -8, -7, -6
Cyclophosphamide	200 mg/kg	50 mg/kg	IV in 1 hour	-5, -4, -3, -2
BACT				
BCNU	200 mg/m^2	200 mg/m^2	IV in 2 hours	-6
ARA-C	800 mg/m^2	200 mg/m^2	IV in 2 hours	-5, -4, -3, -2
Cyclophosphamide	200 mg/kg	50 mg/kg	IV in 1 hour	-5, -4, -3, -2
6-Tioguanina	800 mg/m^2	200 mg/m^2	p.o	-5, -4, -3, -2
Alternative "standard" regimens				
TBI/VP				
Total body irradiation	12–13.2 Gy	2–2.5 Gy (2x/day)		-7, -6, -5, -4
Etoposide	60 mg/kg	60 mg/kg	IV in 2 hours	-3
AC/TBI				
Ara-C	36 g/m^2	3 g/m^2	IV q 12 hours in 2 h	-9, -8, -7, -6, -5, -4
Total body irradiation	12 Gy	2 Gy (2x/day)		-3, -2, -1

(*Continued*)

Table 3: *(Continued)*

Regimen	Total dose	Daily dose	Administration	Days
MEL/TBI				
Melphalan	110–140 mg/m^2	110–140 mg/m^2	IV in 1 hour	-3
Total body irradiation	10–14.85 Gy	2 Gy (2x/day)		-2, -1, 0
Bu/Cy (Tuschka)				
Busulfan	16 mg/kg	4 mg/kg	p.o. q 6 hours	-7, -6, -5, -4,
Cyclophosphamide	120 mg/kg	60 mg/kg	IV in 1 hour	-3, -2
Bu/MEL				
Busulfan	16 mg/kg	4 mg/kg	p.o. q 6 hours	-5, -4, -3, -2
Melphalan	140 mg/ m^2	140 mg/m^2	IV in 1 hour	-1
Intensified regimens				
Cy/VP/TBI				
Cyclophosphamide	120 mg/kg	60 mg/kg	IV in 1hour	-6, -5
Etoposide	30–60 mg/kg	30–60 mg/kg	IV in 2 hours	-4
Total body irradiation	12–13.75 Gy	2–2.25 Gy (2x/day)		-3, -2, -1
TBI/TT/Cy/ATG				
Total body irradiation	13.75 Gy	1.25 Gy (3x/day)		-9, -8, -7, -6
Thiotepa	10 mg/kg	5 mg/kg	IV in 1–2 hours	-5, -4
Cyclophosphamide	120 mg/kg	60 mg/kg	IV in 1 hour	-3, -2
ATG	120 mg/kg	30 mg/kg	IV in 5–6 hours	-5, -4, -3, -2

(Continued)

Table 3: (*Continued*)

Regimen	Total dose	Daily dose	Administration	Days
Bu/Cy/MEL				
Busulfan	16 mg/kg	4 mg/kg	p.o. q 6 hours	-7, -6, -5, -4
Cyclophosphamide	120 mg/kg	60 mg/kg	IV in 1 hour	-3, -2
Melphalan	140 mg/m^2	140 mg/m^2	IV in 1 hour	-1
Reduced intensity regimens				
TBI/Fluda				
Total body irradiation	2 Gy	2 Gy		0
Fludarabine	90 mg/m^2	30 mg/m^2	IV in 30 min	-4,-3,-2
Fluda/Bu/ATG				
Fludarabine	180 mg/m^2	30 mg/ m^2	IV in 30 min	-10 to -5
Busulfan	8 mg/kg	4 mg/kg	p.o. q 6 hours	-6, -5
± ATG	40 mg/kg	10 mg/kg	IV in 8–10 hours	-4, -3, -2, -1

hyperplastic bone marrows, e.g. thalassaemia. Partial engraftment may be sufficient in situations where only a 'specific product' is required, e.g. B-cells in some immunodeficiency states.

Until recently, it was thought that the mechanism of cure of the malignancy was entirely due to the conditioning therapy, and that the HSCT itself was merely a supportive measure designed to allow the patient to receive so-called supra-lethal treatment without experiencing permanent bone marrow aplasia. However, the observation that disease recurrence was more frequent after TCD HSCT identified the 'graft versus leukaemia' effect (GVL). Although GVL is important in the maintenance of remission, this effect cannot be solely responsible for the durable disease-free remission seen in recipients of syngeneic and autologous HSCT. Reduced intensity conditioning (RIC) HSCT has been recently developed in the hope of reducing toxicity and mortality. Its goal is not tumour eradication or destruction of host haematopoiesis by cytotoxic therapy but via immune mediated effects. The immunosuppressive potential of the approach is based on several components: initial conditioning, graft composition, post-transplant rejection prevention and use of donor lymphocyte infusions (DLI) in case of incomplete chimerism at specified time points. Many of these regimens require double immunosuppression with both CsA and MMF post-transplant.

Early Complications After HSCT

The high dose chemo-radiotherapy included in conditioning regimens (see above) affects all organs and tissues, producing early and late secondary effects of variable intensity.

Haemorrhagic cystitis (HC): HC after HSCT can be produced by direct toxicity of the conditioning regimen on the urothelium or by viral infections affecting the urinary tract. Usually, HC due to conditioning appears early after HSCT (several days after receiving CT agents) while viral HC appears later (usually after day +30).[1] The most frequent viruses involved are Human Polyomavirus type BK or JC, Adenovirus type 11 (less frequent) and CMV (exceptional). The incidence of HC related to conditioning without prevention is up to 70% but with prevention with mesna, hyperhydration and sometimes bladder irrigation, it can be reduced to 1% to 25%. The treatment of HC includes forced hydration and aggressive platelet support. In case of clots or vesical pain, then continuous irrigation, IVIG, cystoscopy and removal of clots, selective arterial embolization, suprapubic cystostomy and cystectomy.[34,35]

Early complications of vascular origin: the injury of the vascular endothelium seems to be the most important initial event of several complications with imprecise diagnostic criteria and overlapping clinical features, which are observed within the first 30–60 days after HSCT. The best defined syndromes resulting from this endothelial injury are: sinusoidal obstruction syndrome of the liver, capillary leak syndrome, engraftment syndrome, diffuse alveolar haemorrhage, thrombotic microangiopathy and idiopathic pneumonia syndrome.

Sinusoidal obstruction syndrome (SOS) of the liver is the term used to designate the symptoms and signs that appear early after HSCT as a consequence of the direct hepatic toxicity of the conditioning regimen. This syndrome, formerly termed veno-occlusive disease of the liver (VOD), is characterized by the development of jaundice, fluid retention, weight gain and hepatomegaly, usually painful.[36–43] The pathogenesis is not well known, but the probable succession of events is as follows.[36,37] In the first phase there is hepatic accumulation of toxic metabolites (e.g. acrolein) produced by the metabolism of certain drugs by the cytochrome P-450 enzymatic system and decreased transformation of these toxic metabolites to stable metabolites by an inadequate glutathione enzymatic system (due to previous liver disease or the action of agents such as Busulfan, BCNU or TBI). Toxic metabolites are predominantly located in area 3 of the acinus (around centrilobular veins) because this area is rich in P-450 and poor in glutathione, producing damage of hepatocytes and sinusoidal endothelium. After endothelial damage and the procoagulant events there is a reduction of the hepatic venous outflow causing painful hepatomegaly, postsinusoidal intrahepatic portal hypertension and ascites. Due to unclear mechanisms, this is followed by a reduction of renal excretion of sodium and fluid retention, causing oedema, weight gain and worsening ascites.

The diagnosis is mainly based on clinical criteria.[36–38] The Seattle criteria include two or more of the following in the first 20 days after HSCT: bilirubin >2 mg/dL; hepatomegaly or pain in the right-upper quadrant and weight gain (>2% basal weight). The Baltimore criteria require a bilirubin >2 mg/dL + ≥2 of the following: painful hepatomegaly, ascites or weight gain (>5% basal weight). Other complementary studies include abdominal ultrasound, haemodynamic supra hepatic studies with a HVGP of 10 mmHg or greater and liver biopsy showing the classical changes of VOD such as concentric non-thrombotic narrowing of the lumen of small intrahepatic veins; eccentric narrowing of the venular lumen; phlebosclerosis; sinusoidal fibrosis and hepatocyte necrosis. The treatment is mainly symptomatic with restriction of salt and water intake, diuretics and support of the intravascular volume and renal perfusion by means of albumin, plasma expanders and transfusions (to maintain an haematocrit >30%). Direct measures include defibrotide, low dose dopamine, TIPS (transvenous intrahepatic portosystemic shunt), surgical shunt and, if indicated, liver transplantation.[39,42,43]

The clinical manifestations of the thrombotic microangiopathy associated with HSCT include microangiopathic haemolytic anaemia (MHA) (anaemia, fragmented red cells >5%, increased LDH and other markers of haemolysis), thrombocytopenia or increase in requirement for platelet transfusions, fever of non-infectious origin and renal insufficiency or neurological changes.[44] The incidence is around 10–15% depending on the series and risk factors include use of cyclosporine or tacrolimus, GVHD, infections (CMV, fungal) or prior TBI. Several clinical forms are described:

- Nephrotoxicity due to Cyclosporine A (CsA) with MHA: occurs early after HSCT and is reversible after stopping CsA.
- Neurotoxicity due to CsA with MHA: similar to the previous one but with CNS disturbances (cortical blindness, seizures, typical images in CNS scan). Good evolution if it improves quickly when stopping CsA.
- Haemolytic uraemic syndrome: characterized by renal impairment, MHA, hypertension and thrombocytopenia. Occurs mainly in children and has no relation with high CsA levels. Low mortality and good response to plasmapheresis.
- Fulminating multifactorial: Very early after HSCT and characterized by progressive renal failure, CNS disturbances, hypertension,

MHA, and thrombocytopenia. Quickly fatal, usually no response to treatment

Graft versus Host Disease

The principal complication of allo-HSCT is GVHD, which can occur despite aggressive immunosuppressive prophylaxis even when the donor is a 'perfectly' matched (HLA-identical) sibling. It is a consequence of interactions between Ag-presenting cells of the recipient and mature T-cells of the donor. There is convincing evidence that T-cells contained in the donor graft or subsequently derived from donor stem cells react to host APC, causing target organ damage that is recognized as clinical manifestation of GVHD.[45,46] Donor T-cells are infused into a host that has been profoundly damaged by underlying disease, infections and particularly by the conditioning regimen, all of which result in activation of host cells with secretion of proinflammatory cytokines such as TNF-α and IL-1.[46] As a consequence, expression of MHC Ag and adhesion molecules is increased, thus enhancing the recognition of host alloantigens. The second step of the afferent phase of GVHD is characterized by donor T-cell interaction with host APCs and subsequent proliferation, differentiation and secretion of cytokines. Cytokines such as IL-2 and IFN-γ enhance T-cell expansion, induce CTL- and NK-cell responses, and prime additional mononuclear phagocytes to produce TNF-α.[45] These inflammatory cytokines in turn stimulate production of inflammatory chemokines, thus recruiting effector cells into target organs. The efferent phase of GVHD is a complex cascade of multiple effectors such as CTLs and NK cells, and inflammatory effectors such as TNF-α, IL-1 and nitric oxide (NO). The effector functions of mononuclear phagocytes are triggered via a secondary signal provided by lipopolysaccharide (LPS) that leaks through the intestinal mucosa damaged during the initial phase. This mechanism may result in the amplification of local tissue injury. Finally, the inflammatory response, together with the CTL and NK components, leads to target tissue destruction, via target cell apoptosis, in the transplanted host.[46]

The median incidence of clinically significant (grade II–IV) acute GVHD (AGVHD) is about 40% but ranges from 10% to 80% according to risk factors.[47] By convention, AGVHD develops within the first 100 days of transplant.[48] A maculo-papular rash, often involving the palms and soles usually marks the onset of AGVHD. Lesions may be pruritic and/or painful. The rash then spreads and can involve the entire body surface. As the rash intensifies, it is often associated with papules. In more severe cases, bullae can form and surface areas can desquamate, leading to extremely painful denudation associated with protein loss and risk of super-infection. Liver involvement results in cholestatic hepatopathy, with or without jaundice, in which the cholestatic enzymes are substantially raised whilst the transaminases show only non-specific changes. The clinical diagnosis of AGVHD of the liver is difficult since distinguishing liver impairment due to therapy-associated hepatotoxicity, infection, VOD (SOS) or GVHD is not always possible. Involvement of the GI tract primarily manifests as nausea and green watery diarrhoea. The enteral fluid loss is used as a measure of gut involvement. Severe abdominal pain, bloody diarrhoea and massive enteral fluid losses accompany advanced disease. A variant of mild enteric GVHD involving only the upper GI tract has been described. Symptoms include anorexia and nausea without diarrhoea and this usually responds very well to immunosuppressive therapy.

The overall grade of AGVHD usually predicts the clinical course.[48,49] In general, grade I AGVHD has a favourable prognosis. Grade II is a moderately severe disease. Grade III is a severe, multi-organ GVHD and grade IV is life threatening or fatal (Table 4).

Chronic GVHD (CGVHD) is defined by symptoms occurring afterwards, either *de novo*, or following AGVHD. It is a result of a later phase of alloreactivity. It is well recognized that CGVHD is the main determinant of long-term outcome after allo-HSCT. Similarities in the clinical features of CGVHD and several autoimmune diseases have been observed. The skin is the most frequently involved organ (80%). The clinical manifestations include depigmentation, lichenoid papules and dermal and subcutaneous fibrosis with alopecia. Oral involvement (70%) includes lichen planus, ulcerations, atrophy and dryness. The commonest ocular symptom is also dryness (50%), which may evolve into keratoconjunctivitis sicca. Other clinical manifestations are less frequent, including chronic sinusitis, obliterans bronchiolitis, and weight loss with or without anorexia and chronic diarrhoea, myositis, tendinitis and fasciitis.

Table 4: Acute GVHD grading.

a) Grading system: stage for each organ

Stage	Skin/Maculo-papular rash	Liver/Bilirubin	GI/Diarrhoea
+	<25% of body surface	34–50 μmol/lL	>500 mL
++	25–50% of body surface	51–102 μmol/L	>1,000 mL
+++	Generalized erythroderma	103–255 μmol/L	>1,500 mL
++++	Generalized erythroderma with bullous formation and desquamation	>255 μmol/L	Severe abdominal pain with or without ileus

b) Overall grading system (Glucksberg)

Grade of AGVHD	Degree of organ involvement
I	Skin: + to ++
II	Skin: + to +++ Gut and/or liver: + Mild decrease in clinical performance
III	Skin: ++ to +++ Gut and/or liver: ++ to +++ Marked decrease in clinical performance
IV	Skin: ++ to ++++ Gut and/or liver: ++ to ++++ Extreme decrease in clinical performance

Immune deficiency due to CGVHD itself and/or to its treatment is associated with an increased susceptibility to late infections and an increased risk of late morbidity and mortality.

CGVHD was classified in 1980 by Schulman[50] according to the extent of the disease in 20 long-term Seattle patients. With time, the spectrum of abnormalities observed in CGVH has changed, as a result of earlier diagnosis and greater efficacy of immunosuppressive treatments and as the limitations of this classification system have become apparent.[51] Although it is highly reproducible among transplant centres, the traditional grading system is of limited utility because it does not stratify patients for outcome (Table 5).

Prevention of GVHD involves immunosuppressive therapy and T-cell depletion (TCD). Cyclosporine A (CsA) appeared in the early 80s.[52] In

Table 5: Chronic GVHD grading.

a) Limited

1. Abnormality of buccal cavity with a (+) lip or skin biopsy without other signs of CGVHD.
2. Moderate modification of liver function tests with a (+) lip or skin biopsy without other signs of CGVHD.
3. Less than six papulo-squamous plaques or a limited skin rash or depigmentation <20% of body surface with a (+) skin biopsy without other signs of CGVHD.
4. Ocular dryness (Schirmer ≤5 mm), with a (+) lip or skin biopsy without other signs of CGVHD.
5. Vulvar or vaginal lesions with a (+) skin biopsy without other signs of CGVH.

b) Extensive

1. Manifestations on ≥2 organs with symptoms of CGVHD with a (+) biopsy.
2. Weight loss <15% with a contribute biopsy on any organ.
3. Skin more than defined in limited CGVHD with a (+) biopsy.
4. Scleroderma or morphea.
5. Onycholysis or onychodystrophia with a (+) biopsy on any organ.
6. Fasciitis.
7. Contractures due to CGVH.
8. Bronchiolitis obliterans.
9. (+) liver biopsy and abnormal liver function tests.
10. Gut (+) biopsy.

contrast to the non-specific cytotoxic effect of MTX, CsA was the first molecule that specifically inhibits T-cell proliferation and IL2 production. The limitation of the therapy is mainly due to its nephrotoxicity. Other frequent adverse effects include hypertension, liver cholestasis, tremors, hirsutism and CNS disturbances. The 'gold standard' regimen for the prevention of GVHD was established in 1986, based on a randomized study performed in Seattle.[52] MTX given at a dose of 15 mg/m^2 on day +1 and 10 mg/m^2 on days +3, +6 and +11 (referred to as short course MTX) was combined with IV CsA 3 mg/kg/d from D–1 to D+30 followed by oral treatment until D+180. This combination led to a significant decrease in the incidence and severity of AGVHD and to a significant improvement in the survival, compared to either CsA or MTX alone. This regimen is largely used in patients with 'standard risk' leukaemia and a genoidentical donor. More recently, particularly for patients with high risk factors for GVHD, i.e. in matched unrelated donor (MUD) transplants, new immunosuppressive drugs have been tested. Tacrolimus (Prograf) is an immunosuppressive macrolide lactone which blocks the earliest steps of T-cell activation by inhibiting the calcium-dependent signal transduction pathway. Although the mechanism of action, pharmacokinetics and side effects profile of Tacrolimus are similar to those of CsA, its immunosuppressive potency *in vitro* is greater. Phase II and phase III studies have shown that Tacrolimus in combination with a short course of MTX appears active in preventing AGVHD after MUD transplantation.[53] Mycophenolate Mofetil (Cellcept) is a derivative of mycophenolic acid. It blocks T- and B-cell proliferation and down-regulates expression of adhesion molecules. The efficacy of MMF associated with CsA has been studied mainly after RIC regimen. The major toxicities are neutropenia and gut ulcerations.

T-cell depletion of grafts is an effective method for prevention of GVHD.[54] However, the limitations associated with this method are the occurrence of graft failure and/or relapse. In MUD transplants, several randomized or comparative studies have been performed comparing *in vitro* TCD to CsA + MTX, but so far, it has not been conclusively established whether TCD can improve survival.[15] *In vitro* positive selection of CD34(+) stem cells is the preferred technique for TCD. The CD34(-) fraction that contains T-cells can be frozen, making possible a delayed T-cell add back if indicated. Several studies showed effectiveness of *in vivo* TCD, using ATG or MoAb (Campath, Alemtuzumab) as prophylaxis of GVHD after matched unrelated donor (MUD) transplantation. Unfortunately the strong immunosuppressive effect of this treatment is associated with an increased risk of severe infections and a higher TRM. Randomized studies are needed in order to evaluate long-term disease-free survival (DFS) in large cohorts of patients.

The treatment of GVHD is based on Methyl-Prednisolone, at a dose of 2 mg/kg/d. This treatment, associated with CsA, is given for two weeks, and then tapered slowly if there is a complete response to therapy. The response of acute GVHD to initial therapy is of particular importance for the prognosis. Failure of therapy is usually defined as progression after three days, or no change after seven days, or incomplete response after 14 days. Patients in whom initial therapy has failed will receive a second-line treatment. The rate of partial and complete response to second-line therapy varies from 35 to 70%, but the 6–12 months survival is low because of infectious complications or recurrence of GVHD. Corticosteroid refractory AGVHD have received a variety of salvage regimens, including an association of Tacrolimus and MMF; high-dose Methyl-Prednisolone: 5 to 20 mg/kg; various MoAb, such as OKT3, anti-IL2-receptor (Dacluzumab), anti-TNF-α (Infliximab), ATG and Campath. Unfortunately, none of these therapies has been consistently successful in salvaging patients, pointing to the need for new approaches to improve outcome. The possible efficacy of Sirolimus (Rapamycin) has still to be evaluated.

Various approaches have been developed for patients with CGVHD not responsive to first-line therapy with corticosteroids, including low-dose total lymphoid irradiation, PUVA therapy, extracorporeal photochemotherapy, MMF, Tacrolimus and Thalidomide. All these treatments have been reported to improve clinical manifestations.[55] Long-term treatment with high-dose prednisolone is associated with a high risk for morbidity. Complications prominently include avascular necrosis, glucose intolerance requiring administration of insulin, infections, hypertension, changes in body habitus, cutaneous atrophy, cataracts, osteoporosis, emotional lability, interference with sleep, and growth retardation in children.

Immune Reconstitution After HSCT

Assessment of the host immune status is becoming a key issue in allo-HSCT, especially in the long-term follow-up of these patients, because severe post-transplant infections, relapse or secondary malignancies may be directly related to persistent immune defects. Immune deficiency leading to an increased susceptibility to infections lasts for more than a year. In relation to the occurrence of infections, the post-transplant period is subdivided into different phases. Although infections that occur in the first month mostly result from a deficiency in both granulocytes and mononuclear cells (MNC), later post-engraftment infections are due to a deficiency in MNC subsets, primarily CD4 T-cells and B-cells. T-cell reconstitution has been extensively studied because of the central role of T-cells in mediating both GVHD, evidenced by the reduced incidence of this complication following TCD, and a GvL effect as shown by donor lymphocyte infusions (DLI). DLI may cure 20–80% of patients with post-transplant relapsed leukaemia and lymphoma depending on the type and extent of the disease. This is one of the most important breakthroughs in HSCT in the last years illustrating the powerful anti-leukaemia effect mediated by allogeneic lymphocytes and the potential of immunotherapy in the treatment of malignant diseases.

In transplants performed following myeloablative conditioning regimens, immune reconstitution (IR) will depend upon the ability of the haematopoietic graft to generate *de novo* lymphoid and myeloid lineage cells and on the function of mature cells contained in the graft.[56] Post-transplantation, the different MNC populations reconstitute at different tempos. The first cells to reconstitute (within first 100 days) are those of the innate immune response, granulocytes, monocytes, macrophages and NK cells. In contrast, T- and B-lymphocytes remain severely reduced and their function is impaired for several months or years after HSCT.[56]

B-lymphocytes (CD19+ B-cells) normalize by one year after transplant. B-cell regeneration may be associated with transient appearance of monoclonal or oligoclonal B-cell expansions.[57] After a decline in the first several months after HSCT, levels of specific antibodies to protein Ag frequently encountered after transplantation (e.g. CMV) return to pre-transplantation levels within one year. In contrast, antibodies to protein Ag unlikely to be encountered after HSCT (e.g. tetanus, measles, polio) continue to decline. This supports the recommendation of post-HSCT vaccination. Antibody levels in the first year are affected primarily by pre-HSCT antibody levels in the recipient.[57] A persistent defect in IgA, especially in patients with CGVHD explains mucosal infections of the respiratory and digestive tracts. IgG2 and IgG4 subclasses are also deficient in the case of GVHD, accounting for the increased susceptibility to infections, primarily those due to encapsulated bacteria (e.g. Streptococcus pneumoniae or Haemophilus influenzae). PBSC recipients do not have higher antibody levels than BM recipients. Vaccinations with inactivated or conjugated vaccines should be initiated when CD4 and

B-lymphocyte counts are sufficient to expect efficacy, usually from six months post-transplant onwards.

NK cells are lymphocytes that act early in the immune response against infection and tumour-transformed cells. Based on phenotyping (CD16 and CD56), they are the first lymphocyte subpopulation to be reconstituted in all graft settings, usually within three months.[58] Memory T-cells are the first to expand after HSCT; they may be either of donor origin in the case of a non-TCD BM or, in the case of a TCD, originate from host T-cells that have survived the conditioning regimen.[59] They respond quickly to previously encountered pathogens, are easier to trigger, faster to respond and enter tissues more readily than naive T-cells. They are frequently directed towards periodically reactivated herpes viruses, CMV or EBV, which they keep under control. They constitute the majority of oligoclonal T-cell expansions found in healthy adults, especially in the CD8+ population. They are also less dependent than naive T-cells upon recognition of self MHC-peptide complexes in their survival and expansion in the periphery. Finally, some of these probably account for recognition of host MHC-peptide complexes during GVHD as cross-reactive allorecognition and viral-specific immune responses have been evidenced, at least *in vitro*. In the long term, broad immune responses need the reconstitution of a naive T-cell repertoire able to respond to a broad range of pathogens encountered by the host and to tumour antigens. Reconstitution of this compartment is an ongoing process which requires a functional thymus for the recovery of a complete T-cell ontogeny.[60] As stated above, naive T-cells also seem more dependent than memory T-cells upon recognition of self-MHC-peptide complexes for their survival in the periphery. Therefore, MHC mismatches may be considered detrimental for immune reconstitution in many respects, including impairment in thymic selection but also in the homeostasis of the naive T-cell compartment.

Infections After HSCT

Despite considerable progress in the management of HSCT complications, infection remains an important cause of morbidity and mortality after HSCT. Major advances in the management of infectious complications have come from the understanding of the mechanisms of the complex immunosuppression observed during the first months after transplant, their role of predisposition to given infections, and also from well-designed therapeutic trials.

After allo-HSCT following a conventional (myeloablative) conditioning regimen, the pattern of infections can be divided into three periods: a) aplastic phase following the conditioning regimen until neutrophil recovery, b) a second period from initial marrow engraftment to at least the third or fourth month, which is characterized by cell-mediated immune deficiency with decreased number and function of specific and non-specific cytotoxic cells, and c) a late post-transplantation period from the fourth month onwards where immune reconstitution is mainly influenced by the presence and severity of CGVHD. Most patients have Ig deficiency, particularly of IgG2, which is responsible for a decrease in the response to polysaccharide Ag.

Bacterial infections

Because of the hospital environment and its resistant bacteria, the physical environment of transplant patients is specifically designed to decrease the risk of nosocomial infection. Different measures can be implemented. The easiest is simple reverse nurse barrier isolation including mask, gloves and gowns, and strict hand washing to prevent cross-transmission. The control of room air quality through filtration (HEPA) is the main measure used to decrease the risk of aspergillosis.

The second measure is the prevention of bacterial infection by gut decontamination with oral quinolones and/or non-absorbable antibiotics (neomycin, colistin) and a low-microbial diet.

The third measure is the management of central IV lines. Catheters may be the source of bacteraemia with significant morbidity, and potential mortality. During the neutropenic phase, it is controversial whether a catheter should be left *in situ* if blood cultures have documented a pathogen, except in the case of methicillin resistant *S. aureus*, Candida sp., Bacillus sp. and corynebacterium JK, and any hospital-acquired resistant pathogen, such as *P. aeruginosa* or Acinetobacter sp., where the catheter should definitely be removed.[61]

Fungal infections

Aspergillus is the most worrisome fungal infection after HSCT[62] and also the most common cause of infectious death after allo-HSCT.[63] Reported incidences vary from 5% to 20% of transplants; the most common site is the lung and GVHD is the main risk factor. A first peak of incidence occurs during the neutropenic period, particularly in leukaemic patients who had been previously colonized. A second peak in incidence is seen between the second and third months, in patients with severe GVHD. Aspergillus infection may also occur at any time after transplant, particularly when corticosteroids have been used for prolonged periods. Recurrence may also occur in one-third of the patients with previous Aspergillus infection.[8] New effective antifungal agents decrease mortality. Voriconazole has been shown to improve the survival for patients with aspergillosis when compared to a control group treated with conventional amphotericin B.[64] Echinocandins have been studied in refractory aspergillosis with encouraging results. Despite these improvements, the mortality of aspergillus in allo-HSCT patients remains over 50% in recent series. Polymerase chain reaction (PCR) and galactomannan antigenaemia may detect aspergillus infections early on. Candida infection is rare since the advent of azole prophylaxis and has a similar presentation in transplant patients when compared to other haematology patients, including candidaemia, hepato-splenic candidiasis and pneumonia.

Viral infections

Viral infections are frequent after HSCT. They may be life threatening, especially when affecting lung, liver or CNS. The availability of new antiviral agents and results of comparative trials has allowed a better control of herpes virus infections. However, due to the subsequent decrease in CMV infections and diseases, new viral infections have emerged, especially due to respiratory viruses and adenovirus.

HSV infections are extremely common, due to reactivation in sero(+) patients. The main early manifestation is mucosal lesions, difficult to distinguish from chemotherapy-induced mucositis in the absence of viral documentation. These lesions are painful and may be the portal of entry of bacteria from the gut. Treatment with IV acyclovir is usually effective. Acyclovir resistance is rare in HSCT patients, but this possibility must be considered in case of HSV disease documented during prophylaxis.

CMV disease has historically been a main cause of death in allo-HSCT patients other than in cases with both donor and recipient are sero(-). Considering the evidence that CMV infection usually precedes CMV disease, and considering the poor prognosis of CMV disease, a pre-emptive strategy has been adopted by most units. The quantification of viral load by PCR seems to be important since high levels of CMV DNA are indicators for a higher risk of CMV disease. Although first line pre-emptive strategies have been mainly studied with ganciclovir, foscarnet has been shown, in an EBMT comparative trial, as effective and no more toxic than ganciclovir.[65] Both can be used as first-line treatment of CMV infection, for an initial duration of two weeks. If CMV is still detected after two weeks of therapy, an additional course of two weeks should be given. Cidofovir has been studied only in uncontrolled trials and because of its toxicity profile; its use should be reserved for second line pre-emptive therapy. CMV prophylaxis includes transfusion policies to avoid acquisition of CMV through blood products, especially for CMV sero(-) recipients of sero(-) donors. These patients must receive blood products either from CMV sero(-) donors exclusively, or leukocyte-depleted products.

VZV infections occur frequently after allogeneic HSCT. Primary varicella may be severe. High dose intravenous acyclovir is the therapy of choice.

HHV6 infections after allo-HSCT have been associated with pneumonia, delayed marrow engraftment and particularly with prolonged thrombocytopenia and encephalitis. HHV6-DNA is frequently detected in the blood during the first months after transplant, so that its implication in clinical symptoms is difficult to establish, except in encephalitis when HHV6-DNA is detected in cerebro-spinal fluid.

EBV associated lymphoproliferative disease (EBV-LPD) is a life-threatening complication occurring after allo-HSCT. The monitoring of the EBV viral load by quantitative PCR permits the early detection of EBV reactivation that may lead to EBV-LPD. Recipients of a TCD SCT are at higher risk of EBV-LPD. Pre-emptive therapy of EBV reactivation with

Rituximab has been shown to improve the outcome. The infusion of EBV-specific cytotoxic T-cells has also been studied in high-risk patients with elevated EBV-DNA levels. In the absence of prospective trials, the exact indication for pre-emptive therapy based on EBV-viral load for preventing EBV-LPD is not clearly established, and very much depends on the transplant population.

Respiratory viruses, including respiratory syncytial virus (RSV), parainfluenza virus, rhinovirus and influenza virus, appear to be more frequent than CMV in causing pneumonitis. A prospective study from the EBMT in 1998 showed an incidence of respiratory virus pneumonia of 2.1%.[66] Most cases in this series were due to RSV or influenza A. The mortality of these infections also varies among series, and with the time after transplant and the degree of immunosuppression, but it may be as high as 80% in RSV pneumonia. Few data are available in the literature on the efficacy of antiviral drugs in RSV pneumonia. Due to the risk of spread in the transplant unit, it is important to diagnose these patients very early, and to provide adequate prevention of transmission in the ward.

Adenovirus can be a cause of severe disseminated infections in allo-HSCT recipients. Patients receiving mismatched or UD HSCT, or with severe AGVHD, or with viral isolation from multiple sites, and from blood, are at high risk of developing adenovirus organ involvement. There are currently no established regimens for prophylaxis or treatment of adenovirus disease. A recent retrospective study by the IDWP has showed that cidofovir was effective in ten out of 16 patients with invasive adenovirus disease.[67]

Other infections

Toxoplasmosis occurring after HSCT has been mainly investigated in Europe, due to a higher seroprevalence of the disease when compared to the US.[68] Patients at risk are those who are sero(+) for toxoplasmosis before transplant, irrespectively of donor serology. Blood PCR allows an early detection of toxoplasma reactivation. A recent prospective study from the EBMT on toxoplasma reactivation documented by blood PCR shows a frequency of reactivation of 8%. Most reactivations occur in patients with GVHD, when trimethoprim-sulfamethoxazole has been stopped for side effects, and replaced by aerosolized pentamidine for prophylaxis of *P. jiroveci* (previously *P. carinii*). It is not yet clear whether asymptomatic toxoplasma infection documented by blood PCR should be treated. Pneumocystis jiroveci pneumonia must be prevented in allo-HSCT recipients from engraftment to at least six months post-transplant, even longer in case of prolonged immunosuppression. The best option is trimethoprim-sulfamethoxazole. In case of intolerance, alternatives are dapsone or aerosolized pentamidine.

Post-transplant immunization

Active immunization to tetanus, poliovirus and diphtheria is highly recommended in all transplant populations, due to the usual loss of specific immunity after both auto- and allo-HSCT. This is the only way to allow transplanted patients to have relatively normal immunity to these pathogens. Immunization with live vaccines is classically prohibited in immunocompromised patients. However, transplant patients may require active immunization with vaccines that only exist in a live form, i.e. measles, mumps or yellow fever. The current recommendations form the EBMT are summarized in Table 6.

Indications and Results

Allogeneic HSCT remains the best therapy for the control of many malignant and non-malignant diseases. Table 7 shows the current indications from the EBMT.

Results in children

HSCT represents an attractive option for children with high-risk (HR) acute leukaemia, defined as children who have a low cure-rate expectancy with conventional therapies. The first treatment of choice is HLA identical sibling HSCT. Because 80% of children lack this kind of donor, the pros and cons of alternative approaches must be carefully weighed on a case-by-case basis: auto-HSCT can be used in selected cohorts of children with acute

Table 6: EBMT recommendations for immunizations after allogeneic HSCT.

Vaccine	Allo-HSCT recipients	Auto-HSCT recipients	Time for immunization (months)
Tetanus toxoid	++	++	6–12
Diphtheria toxoid	++	++	6–12
Inactivated polio	++	++	6–12
Pneumococci (23 valent)	+/– (S)	+/– (S)	6–12
H Influenzae	++	+ (S)	4–6
Measles, Rubella (attenuated)	+/– (S, R)	+/– (S, R)	Individual*
Influenza	+	+ (S)	6#

++: Strongly recommended for all patients (benefit >> risk). +: Recommended (benefit > risk). +/–: Individual recommendation (benefit and risk must be weighed in individual cases). S: Might have particular benefit in subgroups of patients. R: Regional variations depending on the epidemiological situation. * Not earlier than 24 months after allo-HSCT. # Season dependent.

Table 7: Indications for allogenic HSCT: EBMT guidelines.

Disease	Disease status	Sibling donor	Well-matched unrelated/1ag related	Mm unrelated/ >1 ag related
AML	CR1 (low risk[a])	CO	D	GNR
	CR1 (intermediate or high risk[a])	S	CO	D
	CR2/CR3/Relapse	S	CO	D
	M3 Molecular persistence-CR2	S	CO	GNR
ALL	CR1 (low risk[a])	D	GNR	GNR
	CR1 (high risk[a])	S	S	CO
	CR2, incipient relapse	S	S	CO
	Relapse or refractory	CO	GNR	GNR
CML	First chronic phase (CP)	S	S	GNR
	Accelerated phase or >first CP	S	S	CO
	Blast crisis	GNR	GNR	GNR

(Continued)

Table 7: (*Continued*)

Disease	Disease status	Sibling donor	Well-matched unrelated/1ag related	Mm unrelated/ >1 ag related
Myeloproliferatie disorders		CO	CO	D
Myelodysplastic syndrome	RA, RAEB	S	S	CO
	RAEBt, sAML in CR1 or CR2	S	CO	CO
CLL	Poor-risk disease	S	S	D
Diffuse large cell NHL	CR1 (intermediate/ high IPI at dx)	GNR	GNR	GNR
	Chemosensitive relapse; CR2	D	D	GNR
	Refractory	D	D	GNR
Mantle cell lymphoma	CR1/CR2/Relapse	D	D	GNR
	Refractory	D	D	GNR
Lymphoblastic and Burkitt's lymphoma	CR1	D	GNR	GNR
	Chemosensitive relapse; CR2	CO	D	GNR
	Refractory	D	D	GNR
Follicular B-cell NHL	CR1 (intermediate/ high IPI at dx	GNR	GNR	GNR
	Chemosensitive relapse; CR2	CO	CO	GNR
	Refractory	D	D	GNR
T-cell NHL	CR1	D	GNR	GNR
	Chemosensitive relapse; CR2	D	D	GNR
Hodgkin's lymphoma	CR1	GNR	GNR	GNR
	Relapse; CR2	D	D	D
	Refractory	D	D	GNR

(*Continued*)

Table 7: (*Continued*)

Disease	Disease status	Sibling donor	Well-matched unrelated/1ag related	Mm unrelated/ >1 ag related
Myeloma	All stages	CO	D	GNR
Amyloidosis		CO	D	GNR
SAA	Newly diagnosed	S	GNR	GNR
	Relapsed/Refractory	S	S	CO

S = Standard of care, generally indicated in suitable patients; CO = clinical option, can be carried after careful assessment of risks and benefits; D = developmental, further trials are needed; GNR = generally not recommended; CR1, 2, 3 = first, second, third complete remission; RA = refractory anaemia; RAEB = refractory anaemia with excess blasts; sAML = secondary acute myeloid leukaemia; [a]categories are based mainly on number of white blood cells, cytogenetics at diagnosis and time to achieve remission according to international trials.

lymphoblastic (ALL) or acute myeloid leukaemia (AML); in another 30–40% of cases, a MUD may be available in a short period of time; finally, the last few years have seen a rise in the use of alternative options, such as unrelated cord blood stem cell donors or HLA-mismatched relatives.

The prognosis of AML in children has significantly improved over the past two decades: with intensive chemotherapy 80–90% of children achieve CR and 30–70% are cured if they receive post-induction chemotherapy.[68,69] HLA identical siblings HSCT in CR1 results in 45–64% long-term survival and is an attractive strategy for children who have an HLA-matched donor. Berlin-Frankfurt-Munster Group (BFM) trials 83 and 87 defined an HR group comprising 68% of patients with a five-year EFS of 30–32%.[70] More recently, the Italian Association for Paediatric Haematology and Oncology (AIEOP) identified, on the basis of cytogenetic findings and poor early response, a HR group with similar results. In these patients there is an absolute indication for HSCT.[71] HSCT in CR1 has proven to be more efficient than chemotherapy alone in most comparative studies, with an EFS ranging from 55% to 72% in children given a sibling HSCT in CR1.[68]

Indications for HSCT for children with acute lymphoblastic leukaemia in CR1 are limited to only 8–10% of children, who constitute a subpopulation of very HR ALL.[72] Most study groups define these patients as having an estimated event-free survival (EFS) of less than 50%. SCT from a sibling cures more than 50% of patients who failed first-line chemotherapy. Studies by the AIEOP show that the EFS of patients after sibling HSCT following an early BM relapse is significantly better compared to patients receiving chemotherapy (33% vs 16%), whereas the difference does not reach statistical significance in patients undergoing HSCT following a late relapse (55% vs 40%).[73]

Severe combined immunodeficiency (SCID) consists of a group of genetic disorders characterized by profoundly defective T-cell differentiation, with or without abnormal B-cell differentiation, which leads to early death in the absence of HSCT. The overall frequency has been estimated at between 1:50,000 to 1:100,000 live births.[74–76] SCID is a paediatric emergency that needs to be treated as soon as possible once diagnosis is confirmed. The treatment of choice is an allo-HSCT which provides the missing progenitor of T-cells and allows a survival rate of more than 90% when carried out shortly after birth.[77–79] In the presence of an HLA identical sibling donor, HSCT can be performed without any conditioning regimen and its course is characterized by the absence of GVHD and by the rapid development of the T-cell function post-transplant. In the European experience (1968–99) for the EBMT/ESID group, three-year survival with evidence of sustained engraftment and improvement of the immunodeficiency disorder was 77% with a significant improvement over time from 62% in 1968–85 up to 82% in 1999.[77]

Bone marrow failure (BMF) syndromes in children group several distinct entities including idiopathic and post-hepatitis SAA that are not very different from the syndrome found in adults and several hereditary disorders which must be excluded before any attempt of treatment. Fanconi anaemia (FA) is a rare autosomal recessive disease characterized by congenital abnormalities, progressive BMF, chromosome breakage and cancer susceptibility. At least nine genes have been involved in the disease, which products functionally interact within the FA/BRCA biochemical pathway. HSCT is currently the only treatment that definitively restores normal haematopoiesis. FA anaemia cells are hypersensitive to DNA cross-linking agents. Cellular exposure to toxic agents including Cy, Bu or irradiation increases chromosome breaks and tissue damage. GVHD induces severe tissue damage and absence of repair. Therefore, standard conditioning must not be used. In a recent series of FA patients, conditioned with low dose Cy and TLI, five-year survival was 85% but the probability of head and neck carcinoma increased with time. The absence of irradiation in the conditioning regimen did not abolish the risk of secondary tumours, which are likely also to be related to the specific genetic defect present and to the environment, as shown by different phenotypic expression of the disease in homozygous twins.[80]

β-thalassemia and sickle cell disease (SCD) represent the most frequent haemoglobinopathies worldwide. Although supportive therapies can ameliorate their symptoms, HSCT represents the only cure for these diseases. In the last few years the outcome of HSCT for haemoglobinopathies has progressively improved thanks to the development of better conditioning regimens and supportive therapies. While the role of HSCT for β-thalassemia has been increasingly better defined, the use of this therapeutic strategy for SCD is still controversial and requires further investigation.[81]

Results in adults

For adult patients with acute leukaemia (AL), HSCT is the treatment associated with the lowest relapse incidence. AL is classified in two groups: acute myeloid leukaemia (AML) and acute lymphoblastic leukaemia (ALL). Both are treated with chemotherapy at the beginning of the disease to induce remission. The treatment plan involves a remission induction phase aimed at establishing a CR and a post-induction phase aimed at eradicating/reducing residual disease. Combination chemotherapy induces CR in an average of 60% to 80% of adults aged less than 60 years. In general, HSCT is performed after two or three courses of CT.

AML patients can be stratified according to three risk groups:[82–84]

1. For good-risk patients in first CR, chemotherapy seems not inferior to transplant strategies. These patients include those with favourable cytogenetics such as t(8;21) and Inv16 and patients with acute

promyelocytic leukaemia (APL, AML-M3), which is characterized by the PML-RARA fusion gene arising from the t(15;17).

2. For poor-risk patients and for all other patients who relapse, the chance of surviving without a transplant is very low. Poor risk includes patients not achieving CR after one or two courses of chemotherapy or patients with unfavourable cytogenetics such as abnormalities of chromosome 3, 5 or 7, 11q23 rearrangements (MLL gene), t(9;22) or complex karyotype. For those patients an early transplant strategy should be organized.
3. The remaining patients, including those with normal cytogenetics are considered intermediate risk. For intermediate-risk patients with an HLA compatible sibling, allo-HSCT remains the best option. However, 30% of patients with no cytogenetic abnormality have an abnormality of the FLT3 gene, either an internal tandem duplication (ITD) or a point mutation. These patients may benefit from early transplantation from the best available donor.

In all studies which have tried to compare chemotherapy with allo-HSCT, allogeneic HSCT has never been shown to be inferior and was often superior.[85–87] However such studies have not so far completely clarified the situation. Patients under 55 in the UK MRC AML 10 trial who entered CR were tissue typed (n = 1,063). Four hundred-and-nineteen had a matched sibling donor and 644 had no match. When compared on a donor vs no donor basis the relapse incidence (RI) was reduced in the donor arm (36% vs 52%; p = 0.001) and the DFS improved (50% vs 42%; p = 0.01), but overall survival (OS) was not different (55% vs 50%). Sixty-one percent of patients with a donor underwent HSCT. A significant benefit in DFS was seen in the intermediate-risk cytogenetic group (50% vs. 39%; p = 0.004). Allo-HSCT given after intensive chemotherapy was able to reduce RI in all risk and age groups. However, due to the competing effects of procedural mortality and an inferior response to CT if relapse does occur, there was a survival advantage only in patients of intermediate risk.[84]

Results with unrelated donors show for patients in first CR, second CR and advanced phase a TRM of 20%, 42% and 48%, a relapse rate of 33%, 29% and 60% and a leukaemia-free survival of 50%, 42% and 28%

respectively.[88] Using Eurocord registry data a matched pair analysis was performed in order to compare the results of UD-CBT versus UD-BMT in adults with AL.[89] The incidence of AGVHD was 32% after UD-CBT compared to 41% after UD-BMT ($p = 0.05$) and the incidence of CGVHD at two years was not statistically different ($p = 0.53$). Kaplan-Meier estimates of transplant related mortality (TRM) at day 100 and two years were respectively 37% and 66% after UD-CBT compared to 27% ($p = 0.08$) and 46% ($p = 0.12$) after UD-BMT. Two-year RI and survival were similar in both groups of patients. These data suggest that despite increased HLA disparities, the probabilities of relapse, OS and leukaemia-free survival (LFS) after UD-CBT are comparable to those observed after UD-BMT. Therefore UD-CBT with a high number of infused cells (>1.0 × 10^7/kg) and no more than two HLA disparities should be considered an acceptable alternative for adults with AL.[89] Haplo-identical transplant has been developed by the Perugia group.[90–93] Their most recent publications report the results in 33 AML patients transplanted with a median age of 38 (9–62). All were at high risk because of relapse at transplant, or second or later CR, or CR1 but with unfavourable prognostic features. Positively selected CD34+cells were used and no post-transplant immunosuppressive therapy was given. Leukaemia relapse was largely controlled in AML recipients whose donor was NK alloreactive, with only two out of 16 relapsing. To date, 13 of 18 AML (72%) who were in any CR at transplant survive disease-free while four of the 15 patients (27%) in relapse at transplant survive. The probability of LFS for patients transplanted in CR was 60% and was significantly better in the 16 AML patients whose transplant included donor vs recipient NK cell alloreactivity (70% vs 7%).

There are only a few comparative prospective trials evaluating the best post-remission therapy for adult ALL patients. In the French LALA87 study, patients aged 15 to 40 who achieved a CR and had a matched related donor were assigned to allo-HSCT.[94,95] The intention-to-treat analysis found an advantage for allografting vs chemotherapy (ten years OS = 46% vs 31%). High-risk patients (Ph(+), age > 35, WBC > 30,000/µL at diagnosis, or time to achieve CR > four weeks) benefited more from allo-HSCT (ten years OS = 44% vs 11%).[95] The MRC UKALL XII/ EGOG 2993 study,[96] which is the largest prospective randomized trial designed to evaluate post-remission therapy in adult ALL, has currently accrued 1,500 patients, including over 1,000 patients with Ph(-) ALL. Ninety-three percent of Ph(-) ALL patients achieved CR. Interim analysis of this study shows a significantly reduced RI in Ph(-) patients assigned to allograft (n = 190), compared with those assigned to chemotherapy (n = 253) (five-year RI = 23 vs 61%, p = 0.001). There was a tendency for improved EFS in all patients assigned allograft, (five-year EFS = 54% vs 34%, p = 0.04), most noticeably in standard-risk patients (five-year EFS = 64% vs 46%, p = 0.05). A retrospective comparative analysis by Horowitz *et al.* (on behalf of the IBMTR) reported the outcome of adult ALL patients (aged 15–45) treated with chemotherapy vs allo-HSCT in CR1.[97] The RI was significantly reduced after allograft compared to chemotherapy (26% vs 59%). However, DFS was not different (44% vs 38%), reflecting the higher mortality rate after allo-HSCT. However, a re-examination of this issue using more recently treated patients demonstrated superior DFS with allo-HSCT for patients < 30 years.[98]

The Philadelphia chromosome occurs in 20–30% of adult ALL patients. Although more than 60% of these patients succeed in achieving CR, most of them will relapse, and less then 10% will remain alive five years after diagnosis. The poor outcome with conventional chemotherapy makes allogeneic HSCT an attractive option for patients with Ph(+) ALL. Dombret *et al.*[99] have recently reported the outcome of 154 patients with Ph(+) ALL who were entered into the prospective multicentre LALA-94 trial from 1994 to 2000. All patients who entered remission and had a matched related/unrelated donor were assigned to allo-HSCT, whereas those without a donor had an autologous HSCT. The existence of a donor and absence of MRD pre-transplantation were both associated with a longer DFS and OS. The ongoing MRC UKALL XII/ECOG 2993 has recently reported the outcome in 167 Ph(+) ALL patients who were treated from 1993 to 2000.[92] As expected, the five-year EFS and OS were higher in the allogeneic recipients, and approached 36% and 42% respectively, compared with 17% and 19% in non-allogeneic transplanted patients.

Final Considerations

Allogeneic haemopoietic stem cell transplantation is a well-established treatment modality in malignant and non-malignant haematological disorders. Years of experience and prospective randomized clinical trials have shown that it can result in cure in a significant proportion of cases. Until a few years ago, this was the main focus of stem cell therapy. However, cellular therapy has experienced a remarkable transformation with the discovery of the functional plasticity of human stem cells. These include haemopoietic stem cells but also stem cells from different origins: embryonic and somatic. Following a phase of excitement and rapid accumulation of results demonstrating the regenerative potential, research in this field is currently undergoing verification studies and prospective phase III trials. This has opened a new era in regenerative medicine.

References

1. Van Beckum DW, de Vries JJ. *Radiation Chimeras*. London: Logos. 1967.
2. Santos GW. Bone marrow transplantation. In *Advances in Internal Medicine*. Ed: GH Stollerman. Chicago: Year Book Publishers. 1979, pp. 157–82.
3. Fabricious Moeller J. *Experimental Studies of Hemorrhagic Diathesis from X-ray Sickness*. Copenhagen. Levin and Munskgaard. 1922.
4. Jacobson Lo, Simmoms EL, Marks EK, Eldredge JH. Recovery from irradiation injury. *Science* 1951;113:510–11.
5. Nowell PC, Cole LJ, Habermeyer JG, Roan PL. Growth and continued function of rat marrow cells in X-irradiated mice. *Cancer Res.* 1956;16:258–61.
6. Mitchinson NA. The colonization of irradiated tissue by transplanted spleen cells. *Br. J. Exp. Pathol.* 1956;37:239–47.
7. Ford CE, Hamerton JL, Barnes DWH, Loutit JF. Cytological identification of radiation chimeras. *Nature* 1956;177:239–47.
8. Billingham RE. The biology of graft versus host disease. *Harvey Lect.* 1967;62:21–78.
9. Gowans JL. The fate of the parental strain small lymphocytes in F1 hybrid rats. *Ann. N. Y. Acad. Sci.* 1962;99:432–55.
10. Main JM, Prehn RT. Successful skin homografts after the administration of high dosage X-radiation and homologous bone marrow. *J. Natl. Cancer Inst.* 1955;15:1023–9.

11. Santos OW, Garver RM, Cole LJ. Acceptance of rat and mouse lung grafts by radiation chimeras. *J. Natl. Cancer Inst.* 1960;24:1367–87.
12. Thomas ED, Lochte HL, Lu WC, Ferrebee JW. Intravenous infusion of bone marrow in patients receiving radiation and chemotherapy. *N. Engl. J. Med.* 1957;257:491–6.
13. Mathe G, Jammet H, Pendic B, *et al.* Transfusions et graffes de moelle osseuse homologue chez des humains irradies a haute dause accidentellement. *Revue Fr. Etud. Clin. Biol.* 1959;4:226–38.
14. Thomas ED, Buckner CD, Banaji M, *et al.* 100 patients with acute leikemia treated by chemotherapy, total body irradiation and allogeneic marrow transplantation. *Blood* 1977;49:511–33.
15. Thomas ED, Buckner CD, Clift RA, *et al.* Marrow transplantation for acute non-lymphoblastic leukaemia in first remission. *N. Engl. J. Med.* 1979;301:597–9.
16. Klein J, Sato A. The HLA system. First of two parts. *N. Engl. J. Med.* 2000;343:702–9.
17. Marsh SGE, Albert ED, Bodmer WF, *et al.* Nomenclature for factors of the HLA system, 2002. *Tissue Antigens* 2002;60:407–64.
18. Petersdorf EW, Gooley TA, Anasetti C, *et al.* Optimizing outcome after unrelated bone marrow transplantation by comprehensive matching of HLA class I and II alleles in the donor and recipient. *Blood* 1998;92:3515–29.
19. Petersdorf EW, Anasetti C, Martin PJ, Hansen JA. Tissue typing in support of unrelated hematopoietic cell transplantation. *Tissue Antigens* 2003;61:1–11.
20. Morishima Y, Sasazuki T, Inoko H, *et al.* The clinical significance of human leukocyte antigen (HLA) allele compatibility in patients receiving a marrow transplant from serologically HLA-A, HLA-B, and HLA-DR matched unrelated donors. *Blood* 2002;99:4200–6.
21. Petersdorf EW, Kollman C, Hurley CK, *et al.* Effect of HLA class II gene disparity on clinical outcome in unrelated donor hematopoietic cell transplantation for chronic myeloid leukemia: the US National Marrow Donor Program Experience. *Blood* 2001;98:2922–9.
22. Flomenberg N, Baxter-Lowe LA, Confer D, *et al.* Impact of HLA class I and class II high resolution matching on outcomes of unrelated donor. *Blood* 2001;98:813a.

23. Weisdorf DJ, Anasetti C, Antin JH, *et al.* Allogeneic bone marrow transplantation for chronic myelogenous leukemia: comparative analysis of unrelated versus matched sibling donor transplantation. *Blood* 2002;99(6):1971–7.
24. Couban S, Barnett M. The source of cells for allografting. *Biol. Blood Marrow Transplant.* 2003;9:669–73.
25. Champlin RE, Schmitz N, Horowitz MM, *et al.* Blood stem cells compared with bone marrow as a source of hematopoietic cells for allogeneic transplantation. *Blood* 2000;95:3702–9.
26. Bensinger WI, Martin PJ, Storer B, *et al.* Transplantation of bone marrow as compared with peripheral blood from HLA identical relatives in patients with hematologic cancers. *N. Engl. J. Med.* 2001;344:175–81.
27. Blaise D, Kuentz M, Fournier C, *et al.* Randomized trial of bone marrow versus lenogastrim-primed blood cell allogeneic transplantation in patients with early stage leukemia: a report from the Société Française de Greffe de Moelle. *J. Clin. Oncol.* 2000;18:537–46.
28. Gorin NC, Labopin M, Rocha V, *et al.* For the acute leukemia working party (ALWP) of the European Cooperative group for Blood and Marrow Transplantation (EBMT): Marrow versus peripheral blood for geno-identical allogeneic stem cell transplantation in acute myelocytic leukemia: influence of dose and stem cell source shows better outcome with rich marrow. *Blood* 2003;102:3043–51.
29. Ringden M, Remberger V, Runde. Peripheral blood stem cell transplantation from unrelated donors: a comparison with marrow transplantation. *Blood* 1999;94:455–64.
30. Remberger M, Ringden O, Blau IW, *et al.* No difference in graft versus host disease, relapse and survival comparing peripheral blood stem cells to bone marrow using unrelated donors. *Blood* 2001;98:1739–45.
31. Ringden M, Labopin A, Bacigalupo, *et al.* Transplantation of peripheral blood stem cells as compared with bone marrow from HLA identical siblings in adult patients with acute myeloid leukemia and acute lymphoblastic leukemia. *J. Clin. Oncol.* 2002;20:4655–64.
32. Rocha V, Cornish J, Sievers EL, *et al.* Comparison of outcome of unrelated bone marrow and umbilical cord blood transplants in children with acute leukemia. *Blood* 2001;97:2962–71.

33. Thomas, *et al.* A history of bone marrow transplantation. In *Thomas' Hematopoietic Cell Transplantation*, 3rd Edition. Eds: KG Blume, SJ Forman, FR Appelbaum. Oxford: Blackwell Publishing. 2004, pp. 4–8.
34. Sencer SF, Haake RJ, Weisdorf DJ. Hemorrhagic cystitis after bone marrow transplantation. Risk factors and complications. *Transplantation* 1993;56:875–9.
35. Gine E, Rovira M, Real I, Burrel M, Montana J, Carreras E, Montserrat E. Successful treatment of severe hemorrhagic cystitis after hemopoietic cell transplantation by selective embolization of the vesical arteries. *Bone Marrow Transplant* 2003;31:923–5.
36. McDonald GB, Hinds MS, Fisher LD, *et al.* Veno-occlusive disease of the liver and multi-organ failure after bone marrow transplantation: a cohort study of 355 patients. *Ann. Intern. Med.* 1993;118:255–67.
37. Carreras E, Bertz H, Arcese W, *et al.* Incidence and outcome of hepatic veno-occlusive disease (VOD) after blood and marrow transplantation (BMT): a prospective cohort study of the European group for Blood and Marrow Transplantation (EBMT). *Blood* 1998;92:3599–604.
38. Lee JL, Gooley T, Bensinger W, *et al.* Veno-occlusive disease of the liver after busulfan, melphalan, and thiotepa conditioning therapy: incidence, risk factors, and outcome. *Biol. Blood Marrow Transplant.* 1999;5:306–15.
39. Carreras E. Veno-occlusive disease of the liver after hematopoietic cell transplantation. *Eur. J. Haematol.* 2000;64:281–91.
40. DeLeve LD, Shulman HM, McDonald GB. Toxic injury to hepatic sinusoids: sinusoidal obstruction syndrome (veno-occlusive disease). *Semin. Liver Dis.* 2002;22:27–42.
41. Carreras E, Grañena A, Navasa M, Bruguera M, Marco V, Sierra J, *et al.* Transjugular liver biopsy in BMT. *Bone Marrow Transplant.* 1993;11:21–6.
42. Or O, Nagler A, Shpilberg O, Elad S, Naparstek E, Kapelushnik J, *et al.* Low molecular weight heparin for the prevention of veno-occlusive disease of the liver in bone marrow transplantation patients. *Transplantation* 1996; 61:1067–71.
43. Richardson PG, Murakami C, Jin Z, *et al.* Multi-institutional use of defibrotide in 88 patients after stem cell transplantation with severe veno-occlusive disease and multisystem organ failure: response without significant toxicity in a high-risk population and factors predictive of outcome. *Blood* 2002;100:4337–43.

44. Daly AS, Xenocostas A, Lipton JH. Transplantation-associated thrombotic microangiopathy: twenty-two years later. *Bone Marrow Transplant.* 2002;30:709–15.
45. Billingham RE. The biology of graft versus host reactions. Harvey Lectures 1966–67;62:71–8. Reddy P, Ferrara JLM. Immunobiology of acute graft-versus-host disease. *Blood Rev.* 2003;17:187–94.
46. Glucksberg H, Storb R, Fefer A, *et al.* Clinical manifestations of graft versus host disease in human recipients of marrow from HLA-matched sibling donors. *Transplantation* 1974;18:295–304.
47. Przepiorka D, Weisdorf D, Martin P, *et al.* Consensus conference on acute GVHD grading. *Bone Marrow Transplant.* 1995;15:825–8.
48. Rowlings PA, Przepiorka D, Klein JP, *et al.* IBMTR severity index for grading acute GVHD: retrospective comparison with Glucksberg grade. *Br. J. Haematol.* 1997;97:855–64.
49. Shulmann H, Sullivan KM, Weiden PL, *et al.* Chronic graft-versus-host disease in man: a clinic pathologic study of 20 long term Seattle patients. *Am. J. Med.* 1980;69:204–17.
50. Akpek G, Lee SJ, Flowers ME, *et al.* Performance of a new clinical grading system for chronic graft-versus-host disease: a multi-centre study. *Blood* 2003;102:802–9.
51. Storb R, Deeg HJ, Whitehead J, *et al.* Methotrexate and cyclosporine compared with cyclosporine alone for prophylaxis of acute graft versus host disease after marrow transplantation for leukaemia. *N. Engl. J. Med.* 1986;314:729–35.
52. Nash RA, Antin JH, Karanes C, *et al.* A phase III study comparing MTX and Tacrolimus with MTX and CsA for prophylaxis of acute GVHD after marrow transplantation from unrelated donors. *Blood* 2000;96:2062–8.
53. Wagner JE, Thompson JS, Carter S, *et al.* Impact of GVHD prophylaxis on 3-year DFS: results of a multi-centre randomized phase II-III trial comparing T-cell depletion and CsA and MTX/CsA in 410 recipients of unrelated donor bone marrow. *Blood* 2002;100:75a–6a.
54. Vogelsang GB. How I treat chronic graft-versus-host disease. *Blood* 2001;97:1196–201.
55. Storek J, Dawson MA, Storer B, Stevens-Ayers T, Maloney DG, Marr KA, Witherspoon RP, Bensinger W, Flowers MED, Martin P, Storb R, Appelbaum FR, Boeckh. Immune reconstitution after allogeneic marrow

transplantation compared with blood stem cell transplantation. *Blood* 2001;97:3380–9.

56. Storek J, Viganego F, Dawson MA, Tineke Herremans MMP, Boeckh M, Flowers MED, Storer B, Bensinger WI, Witherspoon RP, Maloney DG. Factors affecting antibody levels after allogeneic hematopoietic cell transplantation. *Blood* 2003;1001:3319–24.
57. Shilling HG, McQueen KL, Cheng NW, Shizuru JA, Negrin RS, Parham P. Reconstitution of NK cell receptor repertoire following HLA-matched hematopoietic cell transplantation. *Blood* 2003;101:3730–40.
58. Talvensaari K, Clave E, Douay C, Rabian C, Garderet L, Busson M, Garnier F, Douek D, Gluckman E, Charron D, Toubert A. A broad T-cell repertoire diversity and an efficient thymic function indicate a favourable long-term immune reconstitution after cord blood stem cell transplantation. *Blood* 2002;99:1458–64.
59. Roux E, Dumont-Girard F, Starobinski M, Siegrist CA, Helg C, Chapuis B, Roosnek E. Recovery of immune reactivity after T-cell-depleted bone marrow transplantation depends on thymic activity. *Blood* 2000;96:2299–303.
60. Hughes WT, Armstrong D, Bodey GP, *et al.* 2002 guidelines for the use of antimicrobial agents in neutropenic patients with cancer. *Clin. Infect. Dis.* 2002;34:730–51.
61. Marr KA. Epidemiology and outcome of mould infections in hematopoietic stem cell transplant recipients. *Clin. Infect. Dis.* 2002;34:909–17.
62. Unghanss C, Marr KA, Carter RA, *et al.* Incidence and outcome of bacterial and fungal infections following non-myeloablative compared with myeloablative allogeneic hematopoietic stem cell transplantation: a matched control study. *Biol. Blood Marrow Transplant.* 2002;8(9):512–20.
63. Herbrecht R, Denning DW, Patterson TF, *et al.* Voriconazole *versus* Amphotericin B for primary therapy of invasive aspergillosis. *New Engl. J. Med.* 2002;347(6):408–15.
64. Reusser P, Einsele H, Lee J, *et al.* Randomized multicenter trial of foscarnet versus ganciclovir for pre-emptive therapy of cytomegalovirus infection after allogeneic stem cell transplantation. *Blood* 2002;99(4):1159–64.
65. Ljungman P, Ward KN, Crooks BNA, *et al.* Respiratory virus infections after stem cell transplantation. A prospective study from the Infectious Diseases Working Party of the European Group for Blood and Marrow Transplantation. *Bone Marrow Transplant.* 2001;28:479–84.

66. Ljungman P, Ribaud P, Eyrich M, *et al.* Cidofovir for adenovirus infection after allogeneic stem cell transplantation (SCT). A retrospective survey of the Infectious Diseases Working Party of the European Group for Blood and Marrow Transplantation. *Bone Marrow Transplant.* 2003;31(6):481–6.
67. Martino R, Maertens J, Bretagne S, *et al.* Toxoplasmosis after hematopoietic stem cell transplantation. A study by the European Group for Blood and Marrow Transplantation Infectious Diseases Working Party. *Clin. Infect. Dis.* 2000;31(5):1188–94.
68. Woods WG ,Neudorf S, Gold S, *et al.* A comparison of allogeneic bone marrow transplantation, autologous bone marrow transplantation, and aggressive chemotherapy in children with acute myeloid leukaemia in remission: a report from the Children's Cancer Group. *Blood* 2001;97:56–62.
69. Creutzig U, Ritter J, Schellong G. For the AML-BFM Study Group: Identification of two risk groups in childhood acute myelogenous leukemia after therapy intensification in study AML-BFM-83 compared with study AML-BFM-78. *Blood* 1990;75:1932–40.
70. Locatelli F, Labopin M, Ortega J, *et al.* Factors influencing outcome and incidence of long-term complications in children who underwent autologous stem cell transplantation for acute myeloid. *Blood* 2003;15(101):1611–9.
71. Schiappe M. Very high-risk childhood ALL: results from recent ALL-BFM trials intergroup studies. *BMT* 2002;30(1):S16.
72. Uderzo C, Valsecchi MG, Bacigalupo A, *et al.* Treatment of childhood acute lymphoblastic leukemia in second remission with allogeneic bone marrow transplantation and chemotherapy: ten-year experience of the Italian Bone Marrow Transplantation Group and the Italian Pediatric Hematology Oncology Association. *J. Clin. Oncol.* 1995;13:352–8.
73. Fischer A, Cavazzana-Calvo M, De Saint-Basile G. Naturally occurring primary deficiencies of the immune system. *Ann. Rev. Immunol.* 1997;15:93–124.
74. Buckley R. Primary immunodeficiency diseases: dissector of the immunosystem. *Immunol. Rev.* 2002;185:206–19.
75. Candotti F, Notarangelo L, Visconti R. Molecular aspects of primary immunodeficiencies: lessons from cytokine and other signalling pathways. *J. Clin. Invest.* 2002;109:1261–9.
76. Antoine C, Muller S, Cant A. Long-term survival and transplantation of haematopoietic stem cells for immunodeficiencies: report of the European experience 1968–1999. *Lancet* 2003;361:553–60.

77. Buckley RH, Schiff SE, Schiff RI. Hematopoietic stem-cell transplantation for the treatment of severe combined immunodeficiency. *N. Engl. J. Med.* 1999;340:508–16.
78. Bertrand Y, Landais P, Friedrich W. Influence of severe combined immunodeficiency phenotype on the outcome of HLA non-identical, T-cell depleted bone marrow transplantation: a retrospective European survey from the European group for bone marrow transplantation and the European society for immunodeficiency. *J. Pediatr.* 1999;134:740–8.
79. Guardiola P, Pasquini R, Dokal I, *et al.* Outcome of 69 allogeneic stem cell transplants for Fanconi anemia using HLA-matched unrelated donors: a study of the European Group for Blood and Marrow Transplantation. *Blood* 2000;95:422–9.
80. Gaziev D. Stem cell transplantation for hemoglobinopathies. *Curr. Opin. Pediatr.* 2003;15:24–31.
81. Burnett AK. Current controversies: which patients with acute myeloid leukaemia should receive a bone marrow transplantation? — An adult treater's view. *Br. J. Haematol.* 2002;118:357–64.
82. Burnett AK, Wheatley K, Goldstone AH, Stevens RF, Hann IM, Rees JH, Harrison G. Medical Research Council Adult and Paediatric Working Parties. The value of allogeneic bone marrow transplant in patients with acute myeloid leukaemia at differing risk of relapse: results of the UK MRC AML 10 trial. *Br. J. Haematol.* 2002;118:385–400.
83. Lowenberg B, Downing JR, Burnett A. Acute myeloid leukaemia. *N. Engl. J. Med.* 1999;341:1051–62.
84. Suciu S, Mandelli F, de Witte T, *et al.* Allogeneic compared with autologous stem cell transplantation in the treatment of patients younger than 46 years with acute myeloid leukaemia (AML) in first complete remission (CR1): an intention-to-treat analysis of the EORTC/GIMEMAAML-10 trial. *Blood* 2003;102(4):1232–40.
85. Zittoun RA, Mandelli F, Willemze R, *et al.* Autologous or allogeneic bone marrow transplantation compared with intensive chemotherapy in acute myelogenous leukaemia. *N. Engl. J. Med.* 1995;332:217–23.
86. Burnett AK, Goldstone AH, Stevens R, *et al.* Randomized comparison of addition of autologous bone-marrow transplantation to intensive chemotherapy for acute myeloid leukaemia in first remission: results of MRC AML 10 trial. *Lancet* 1998;351:700–8.

87. Anasetti C. Advances in unrelated donor hematopoietic cell transplantation. *Haematologica* 2003;88:246–9.
88. Grewal SS, Barker JN, Davies SM, Wagner JE .Unrelated donor hematopoietic cell transplantation: marrow or umbilical cord blood? *Blood* 2003;101:4233–44.
89. Rocha V, Cornish J, Sievers EL, *et al.* Comparison of outcomes of unrelated bone marrow and umbilical cord blood transplants in children with acute leukaemia. *Blood* 2001;97:2962–71.
90. Ruggeri L, Capanni M, Urbani E, *et al.* Effectiveness of donor natural killer cell alloreactivity in mismatched hematopoietic transplants. *Science* 2002;295:2097–100.
91. Ruggeri L, Capanni M, Casucci M, *et al.* Role of natural killer cell alloreactivity in HLA-mismatched hematopoietic stem cell transplantation. *Blood* 1999;94:333–9.
92. Aversa F, Tabilio A, Velardi A, *et al.* Treatment of high-risk acute leukaemia with T-cell-depleted stem cells from related donors with one fully mismatched HLA haplotype. *N. Engl. J. Med.* 1998;339:1186–93.
93. Sebban C, Lepage E, Vernant JP, *et al.* Allogeneic bone marrow transplantation in adult acute lymphoblastic leukaemia in first complete remission: a comparative study. French Group of Adult Acute Lymphoblastic Leukaemia. *J. Clin. Oncol.* 1994;12:2580–7.
94. Thiebaut A, Vernant JP, Degos L, *et al.* Adult acute lymphoblastic leukaemia study testing chemotherapy and autologous and allogeneic transplantation. A follow-up report of the french protocol LALA 87. *Hematol. Oncol. Clin. North Am.* 2000;14:1353–66.
95. Avivi I, Rowe JM, Goldstone AH. Stem cell transplantation in adult ALL patients. *Best Pract. Res. Clin. Haematol.* 2003;15:653–74.
96. Horowitz MM, Messerer D, Hoelzer D, *et al.* Chemotherapy compared with bone marrow transplantation for adults with lymphoblastic leukaemia in first remission. *Ann. Intern. Med.*1991;115:13–8.
97. Oh H, Gale RP, Zhang M-J, *et al.* Chemotherapy vs HLA-identical sibling bone marrow transplants for adults with acute lymphoblastic leukaemia in first remission. *Bone Marrow Transplant.* 1998;22:253–7.
98. Dombret H, Gabert J, Boiron JM, *et al.* Outcome of treatment in adults with Philadelphia chromosome-positive acute lymphoblastic leukemia — results of the prospective multicenter LALA-94 trial. *Blood* 2002;100(7):2357–66.

Index

www.ingramcontent.com/pod-product-compliance
Lightning Source LLC
Chambersburg PA
CBHW050600190326
41458CB00007B/2110
* 9 7 8 1 8 4 8 1 6 4 9 7 0 *